CLASSIC AMERICAN AMBULANCES 1900 THROUGH 1979

PHOTO ARCHIVE

Walt McCall & Tom McPherson

Iconografix
Photo Archive Series

Iconografix
PO Box 446
Hudson, Wisconsin 54016 USA

Library of Congress Card Number: 98-75268

ISBN 1-882256-94-8

99 00 01 02 03 04 05 5 4 3 2 1

Printed in the United States of America

Cover and book design by Shawn Glidden
Edited by Dylan Frautschi

Iconografix Inc. exists to preserve history through the publication of notable photographic archives and the list of titles under the Iconografix imprint is constantly growing. Transportation enthusiasts should be on the Iconografix mailing list and are invited to write and ask for a catalog, free of charge.

Authors and editors in the field of transportation history are invited to contact the Editorial Department at Iconografix, Inc., PO Box 446, Hudson, WI 54016. We require a minimum of 120 photographs per subject. We prefer subjects narrow in focus, e.g., a specific model, railroad, or racing venue. Photographs must be of high-quality, suited to large format reproduction.

PREFACE

The histories of machines and mechanical gadgets are contained in the books, journals, correspondence, and personal papers stored in libraries and archives throughout the world. Written in tens of languages, covering thousands of subjects, the stories are recorded in millions of words.

Words are powerful. Yet, the impact of a single image, a photograph or an illustration, often relates more than dozens of pages of text. Fortunately, many of the libraries and archives that house the words also preserve the images.

In the *Photo Archive Series,* Iconografix reproduces photographs and illustrations selected from public and private collections. The images are chosen to tell a story—to capture the character of their subject. Reproduced as found, they are accompanied by the captions made available by the archive.

The Iconografix *Photo Archive Series* is dedicated to young and old alike, the enthusiast, the collector and anyone who, like us, is fascinated by "things" mechanical.

Dedication & Acknowledgments

The photographs used in this book came from the personal collection of Walter M. P. McCall. Many of these photos were acquired over the years from close personal friend and fellow professional car historian Thomas A. McPherson. Also providing photos were: Matthew B. Lee, Plymouth MI; Steven B. Loftin, Clinton, OK, and Jack Lister, St. Louis, MO. The authors are also grateful to *The Professional Car Society*, an international organization dedicated to the preservation and appreciation of antique and vintage funeral cars, ambulances and related vehicles.

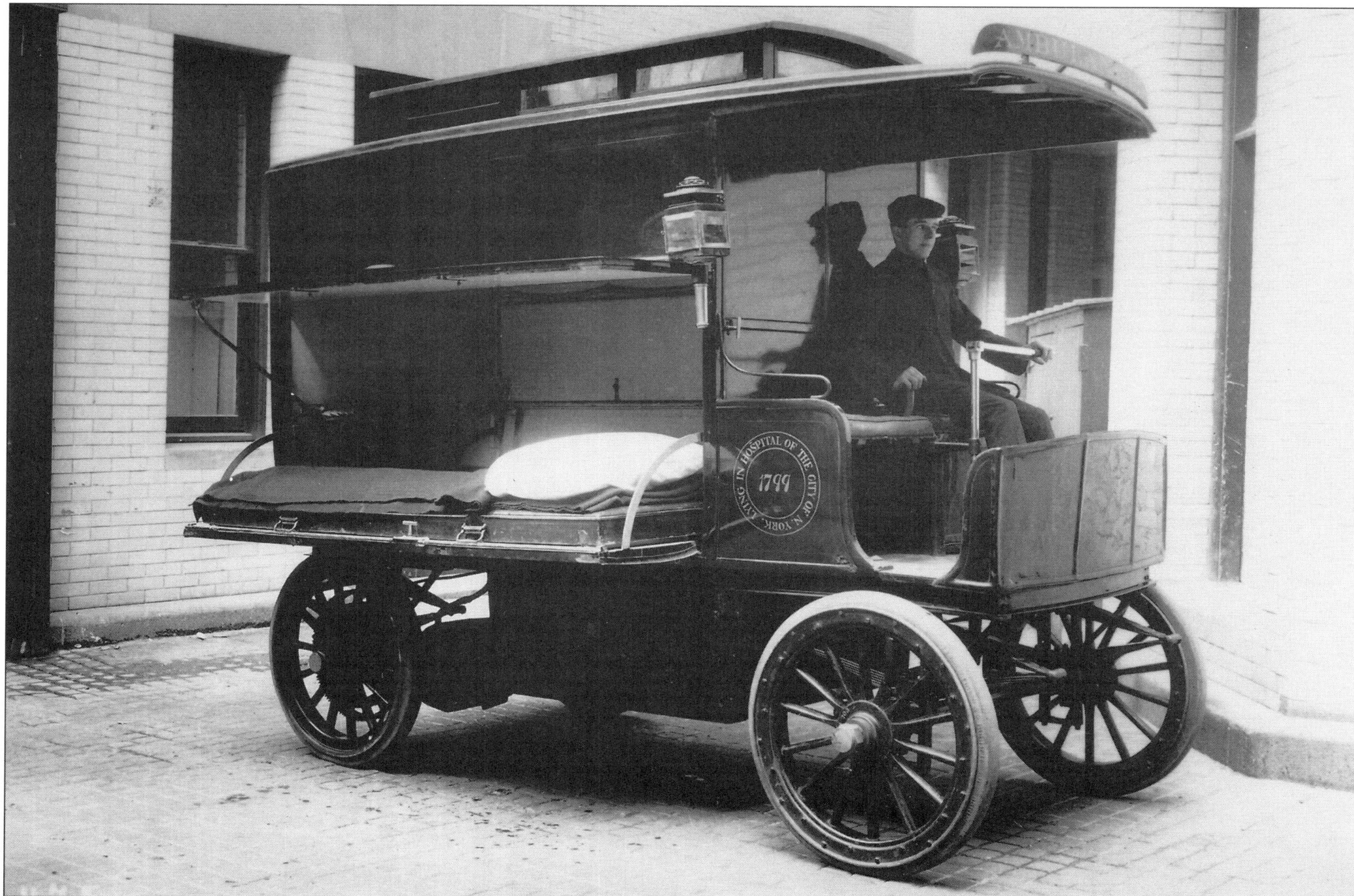

1900 ELECTRIC AMBULANCE - The first automobile ambulances used in the United States were electrics. In the early 1900s, St. Vincent's Hospital in New York City placed in service a battery-powered ambulance built by the F. R. Wood Co. of New York. The Lying-In Hospital of New York placed this side-loading electric ambulance in service on March 1,1900. By 1906, five electric ambulances were silently plying the streets of New York City on their life-saving missions.

Introduction

Speeding through dark city streets, lights flashing and siren screaming, the ambulance on its urgent mission of mercy epitomizes the automobile's most noble public service calling. It is impossible to calculate the millions of lives saved as the result of a speedy trip to the hospital, and the emergency first aid rendered on the way.

For all but the final two decades of the twentieth century, the typical American ambulance was a much-modified derivative of a standard passenger car. Following the demise of the dignified, but woefully slow and inefficient horse-drawn ambulance, the remarkably fast new Auto Ambulance was built on an extended passenger car or light truck frame. By the mid-1920s most of the ambulances being built in North America were constructed on lengthened passenger car chassis with instantly recognizable automobile styling and identity.

As ironic as it may seem today, passenger car-type ambulances were actually a profitable sideline of the closely related funeral car industry. From the birth of the motor ambulance in 1909 through the 1970s - a span of precisely 70 years - the U.S. funeral car and ambulance industries were virtually one and the same. All of the major American ambulance manufacturers were primarily hearse builders: Superior Coach Corp. of Lima, Ohio; A.J.Miller Co. of Bellefontaine, Ohio; Meteor Motor Car Co. of Piqua, Ohio (which later merged to form Miller-Meteor); Sayers & Scovill/ Hess & Eisenhardt of Cincinnati, Ohio; The Flxible Co. of Loudonville, Ohio; The Eureka Company of Rock Falls, Illinois; and Henney Motor Company of Freeport, Illinois.

The same held true for the smaller builders: National, Barnette, Memphian, Comet, Cotner/Bevington and Siebert. Large or small, all of these companies had one thing in common - their principal products were funeral coaches. The ambulances they built utilized the same basic body shell used for their funeral cars. It was a logical and highly successful practice.

For most of this century the local funeral director provided ambulance service to his community on a goodwill basis. In larger cities and towns the funeral director maintained two special-purpose vehicles — a hearse *and* an emergency ambulance. But small town undertakers couldn't afford two separate vehicles. The solution was a single vehicle which could perform both functions, serving as a dignified funeral coach and, by the addition of demountable equipment, as an ambulance as needed. The dual-purpose Combination Funeral Coach/Ambulance was a staple product of the U.S. hearse and ambulance industry for much of the first three-quarters of this century.

As reflected by the photographs in this book, most American ambulances and funeral cars were built on luxury car chassis. Besides utilizing premium quality heavy-duty components, luxury cars depreciated much more slowly and retained their resale value far longer than plebian Fords and Chevrolets. The operator could recoup a significant part of his investment when it came time to trade his hearse or ambulance in on a new one every three or four years.

Improvements were introduced regularly. Luxury ambulances of the 1920s were equipped with hot and cold running water and wicker bassinets for transporting infants. Long, low limousine styling appeared in the mid-1920s; air conditioning in the late 1930s. Raised-roof rescue ambulances could comfortably transport as many as four patients at a time. Other advances included on-board oxygen equipment, two-way radios and quantum leaps in sirens and warning lights.

But the most dramatic change in American ambulance design occurred in the late 1970s. In response to stringent new federal fuel economy standards, the U.S. auto industry "downsized" its products in 1977. At about the same time, new federal ambulance design regulations all but outlawed the soft-riding, passenger car-based ambulance. The first to go was the venerable Combination. Operators could no longer use the same vehicle for funeral and ambulance service.

Downsizing had an immediate and devastating effect on the professional car industry. Cadillac ambulance production plunged to a trickle in 1977. The next two years were even worse. As 1980 dawned, the passenger car-based ambulance had completely disappeared, replaced by much roomier and more efficient van conversions and modular ambulance bodies mounted on light-duty truck chassis.

White-and-Omaha Orange Advanced Life Support Units, manned by highly-trained emergency medical technicians and paramedics, long ago replaced the passenger car-based ambulances which were once a familiar sight on the streets of North American cities and towns. Today's EMT can only wonder what it must have been like to drive and tend patients in those glamorous Cadillacs, Packards and Buicks.

Fortunately, however, there's a happy ending to this story. Many classic American ambulances have been saved and preserved by members of The Professional Car Society. Founded in 1976, this non-profit historical and educational society is dedicated to the preservation and appreciation of antique and vintage ambulances, hearses and related vehicles built off passenger car tooling. For membership information, contact The Professional Car Society, P.O. Box 09636, Columbus, Ohio, 43209, U.S.A.

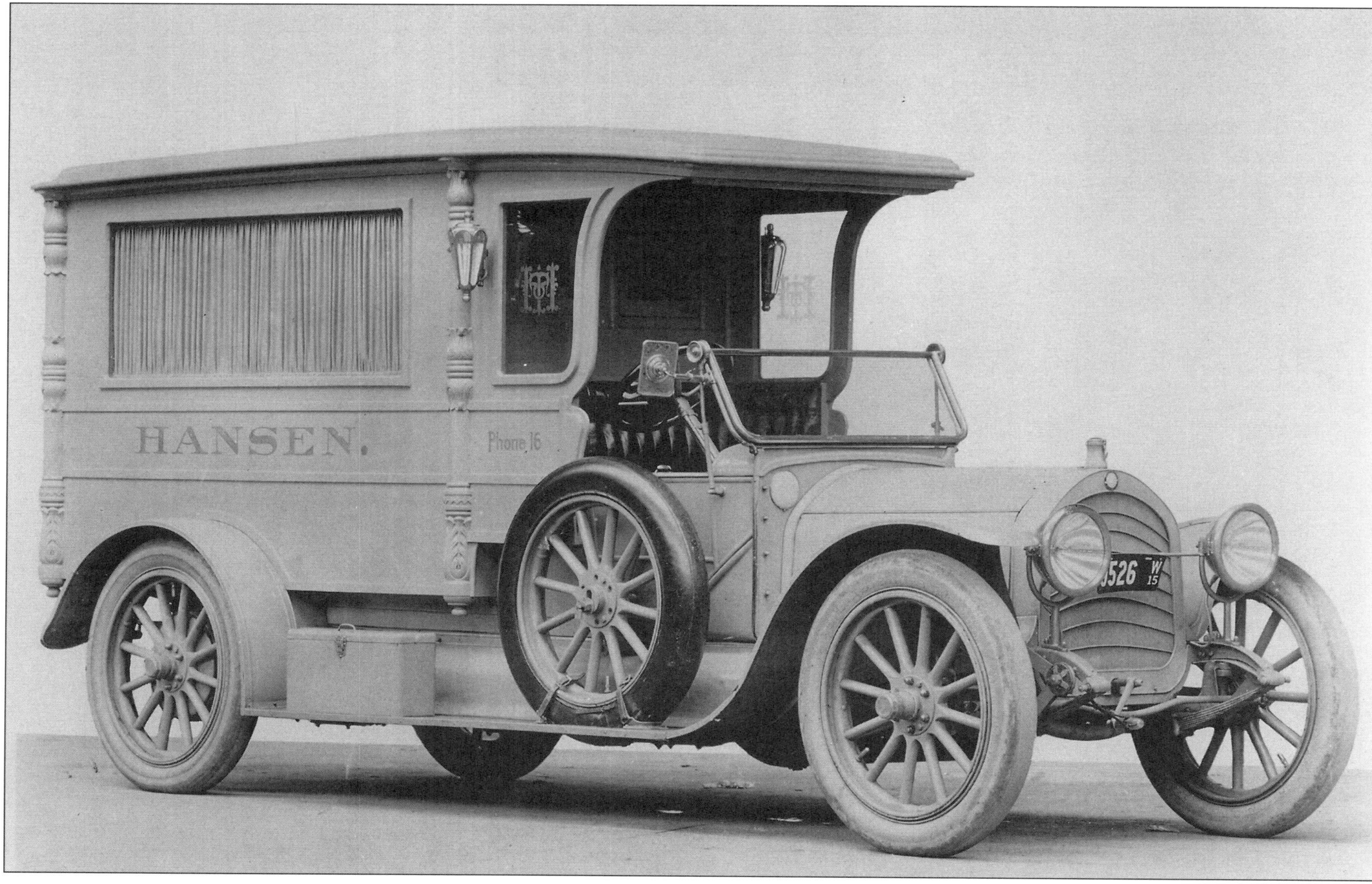

1915 JEFFERY AMBULANCE - The first production gasoline automobile ambulance was introduced by the James Cunningham Son & Co. of Rochester, New York, early in 1909. Within a few years all of America's hearse and ambulance manufacturers had added motor ambulances to their product lines. Into the 'teens,' most of these were of the open-front "C" cab style shown here. This four-column ambulance body is mounted on a 1915 Jeffery chassis built by the Thomas B. Jeffery Co. of Kenosha, Wisconsin. The body builder is unknown, but it could be Seaman.

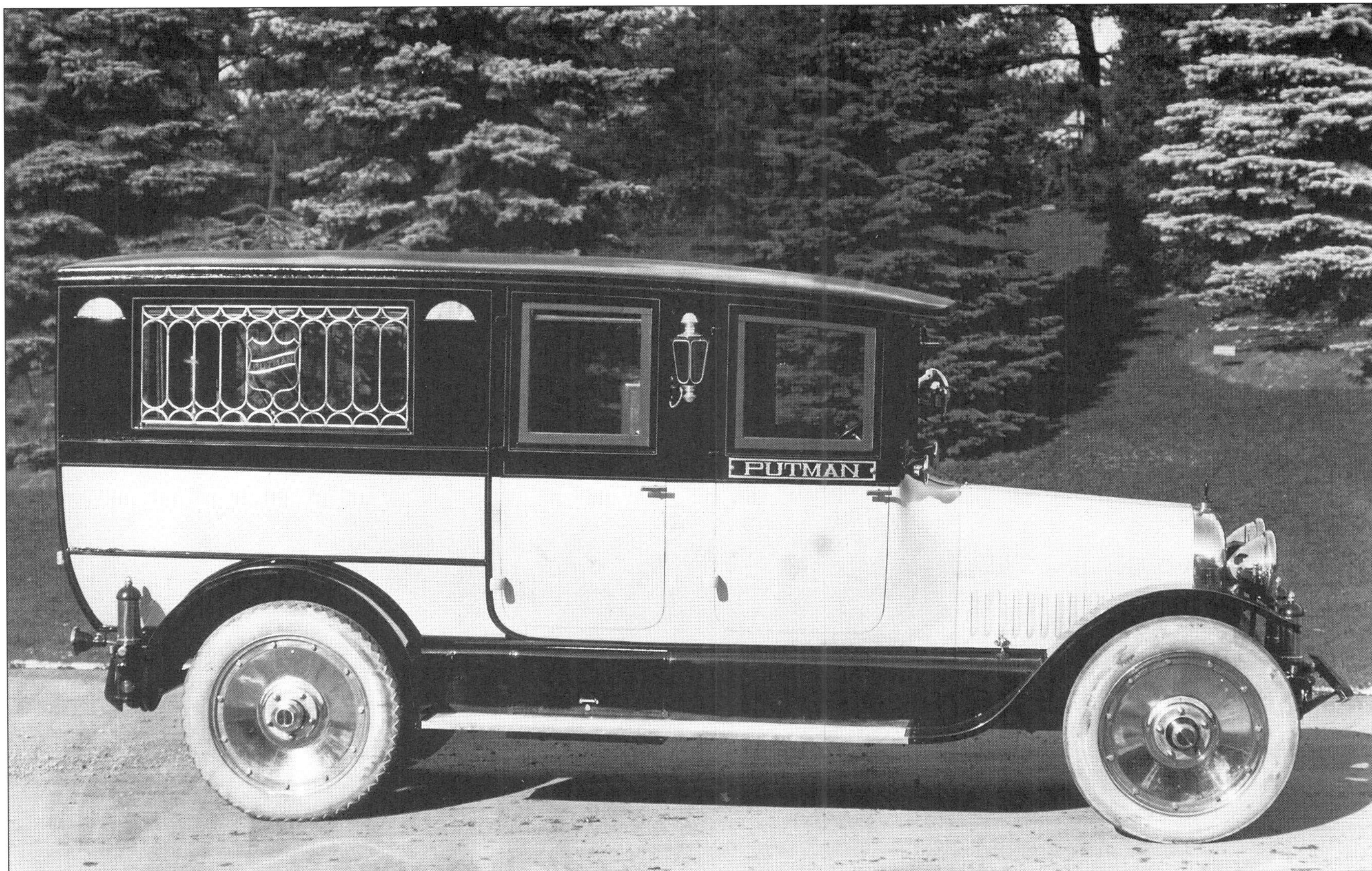

1919 CUNNINGHAM STYLE 68A MOTOR AMBULANCE - Founded in 1838, the prestigious carriage-making firm of James Cunningham Son & Co. of Rochester, New York, entered the automobile market early in the new century. While the company was best known for its superbly engineered luxury cars, Cunningham's bread-and-butter products were premium hearses and ambulances. Note the side-entrance door, leaded windows, elegant carriage lamps and polished disc wheels on this luxury ambulance built on the Cunningham V3 chassis.

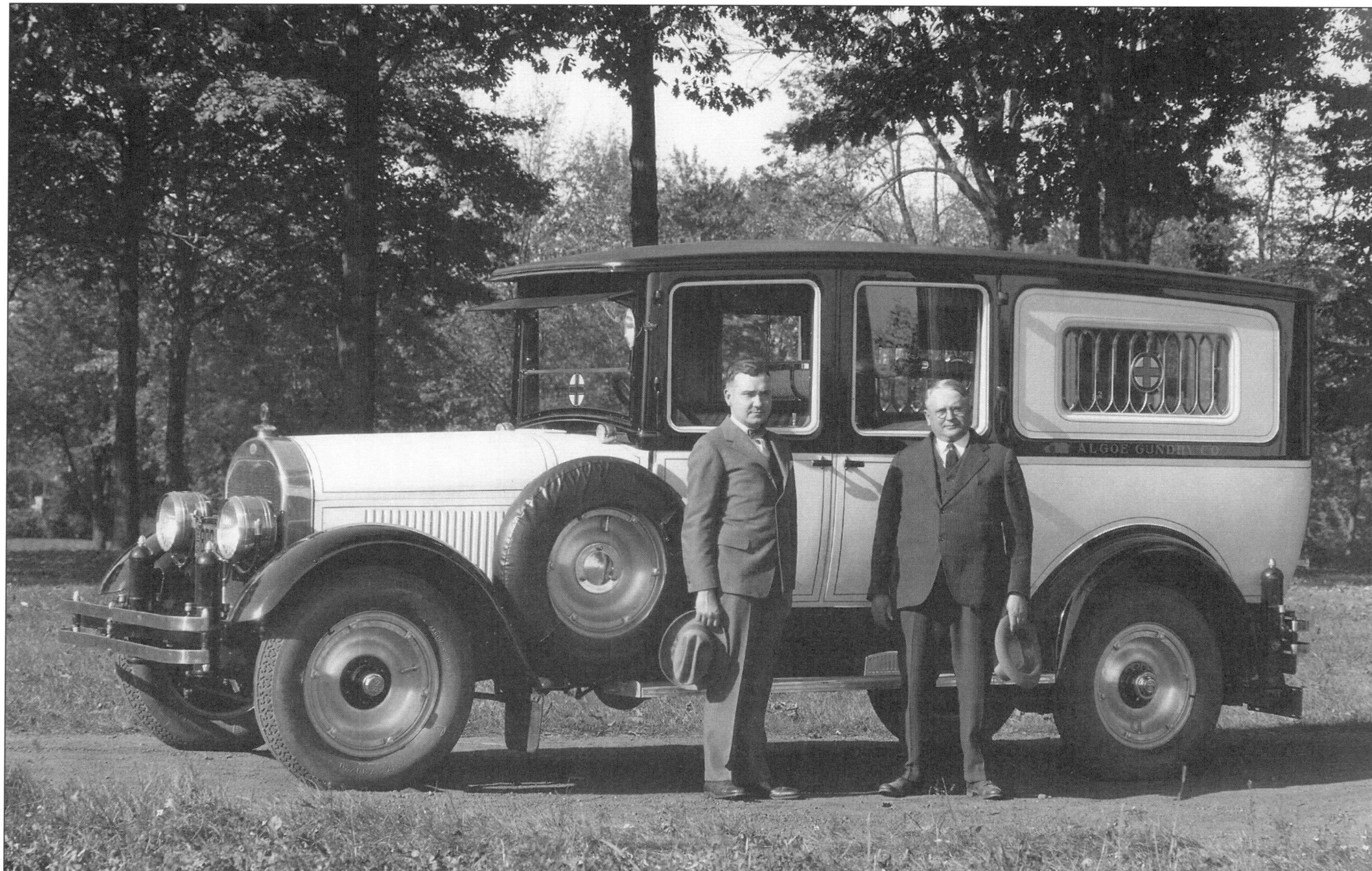

1923 SAYERS & SCOVILL "KENSINGTON" AMBULANCE - One of America's oldest and best-known hearse and ambulance builders was Sayers & Scovill of Cincinnati, Ohio. Founded in 1876, Sayers & Scovill was sold to Hess & Eisenhardt in 1945. The S&S name continues to this day on premium hearses built by S&S/Superior Coaches of Lima, Ohio. Sayers & Scovill built this imposing S&S Kensington Ambulance for the Algoe-Gundry Co. Funeral Directors of Flint, Michigan. The two men standing beside it give a good idea of how *tall* ambulances of this vintage were!

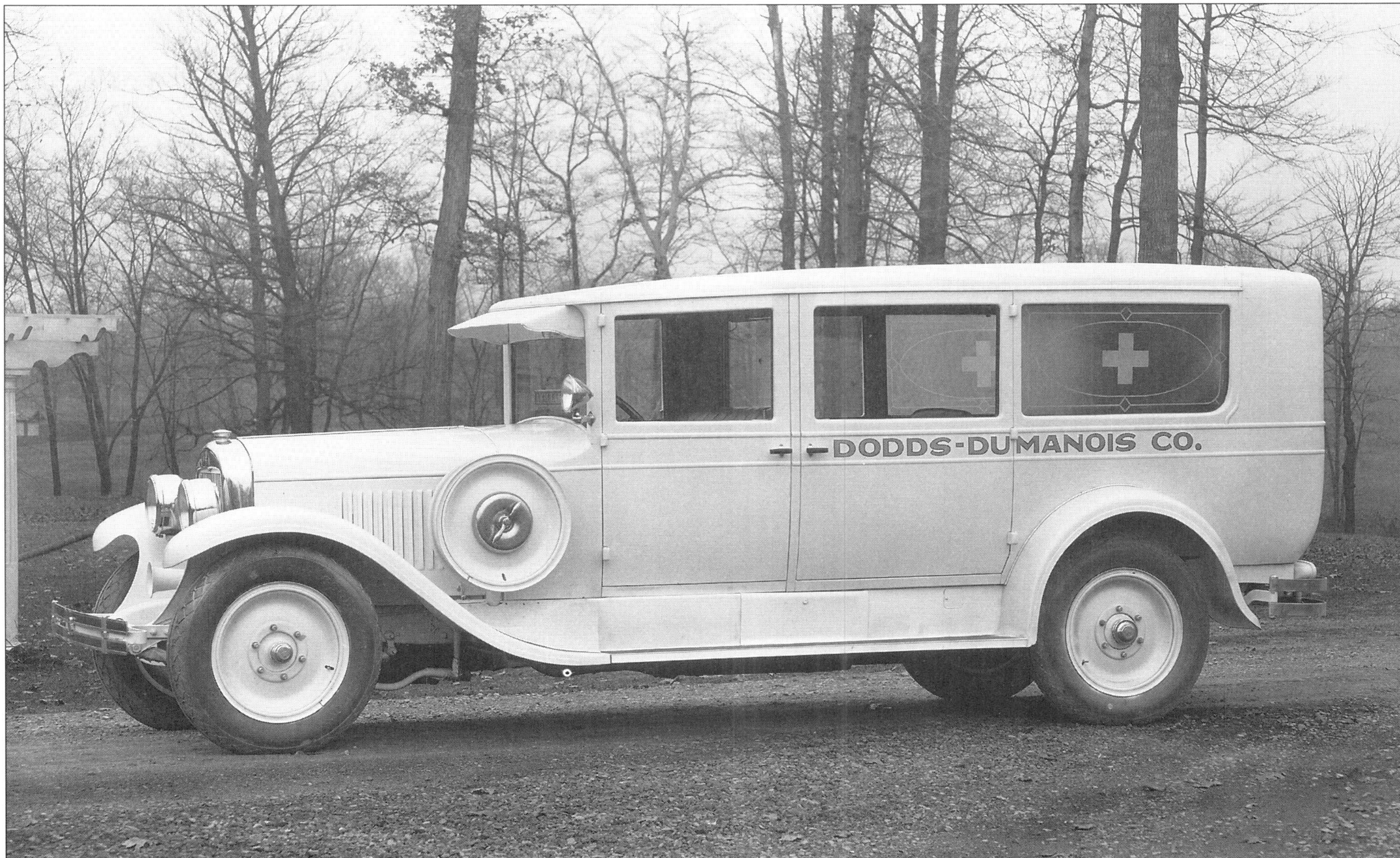

1926 SUPERIOR-CADILLAC LIMOUSINE AMBULANCE - Ambulance and hearse design underwent a dramatic change with the introduction of "limousine" styling in the mid-1920s. The tall, boxy hearses and ambulances which had made the transition from horses to gasoline power were supplanted by long, low limousine style bodies designed to emulate the finest passenger cars of the day. Founded as a bus builder in 1923, the Superior Body Co. of Lima, Ohio, added hearses and ambulances to its product line in 1925. Superior is still in business today, more than three-quarters of a century later.

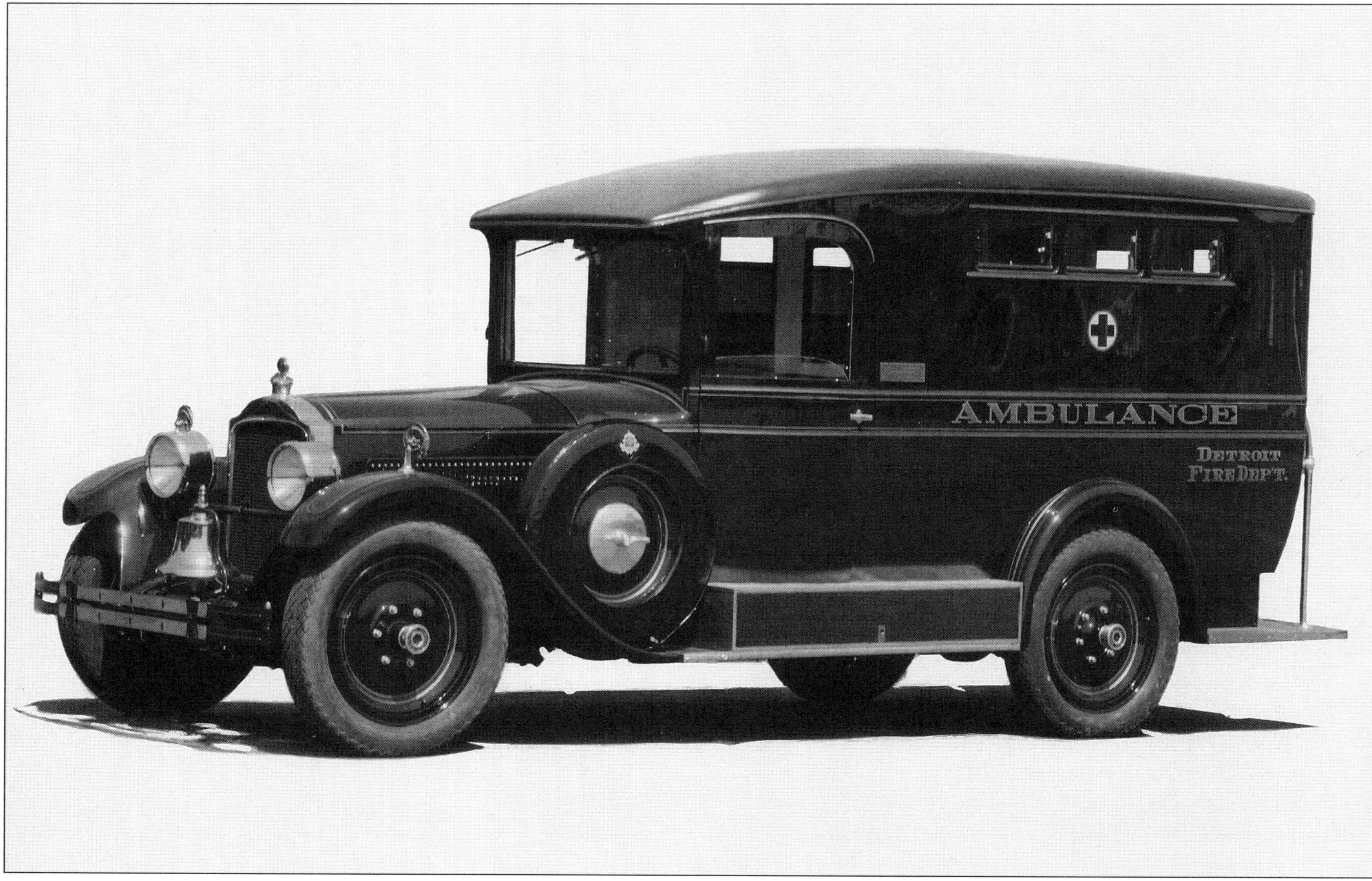

1927 PACKARD AMBULANCE/COMMISSARY - Detroit Fire Commissioner Paxton Mendelssohn presented this combination Ambulance & Commissary to the Detroit Fire Department as a gift in 1927. Mounted on a six-cylinder Packard Model 6-433 chassis, the body was built by Dietrich. Note the front-mounted bell and equipment box on the running board. Replaced by a Cadillac V-16 ambulance ten years later, the 1927 Packard was converted into a floodlight car. Retired in 1948, it is still on the road today.

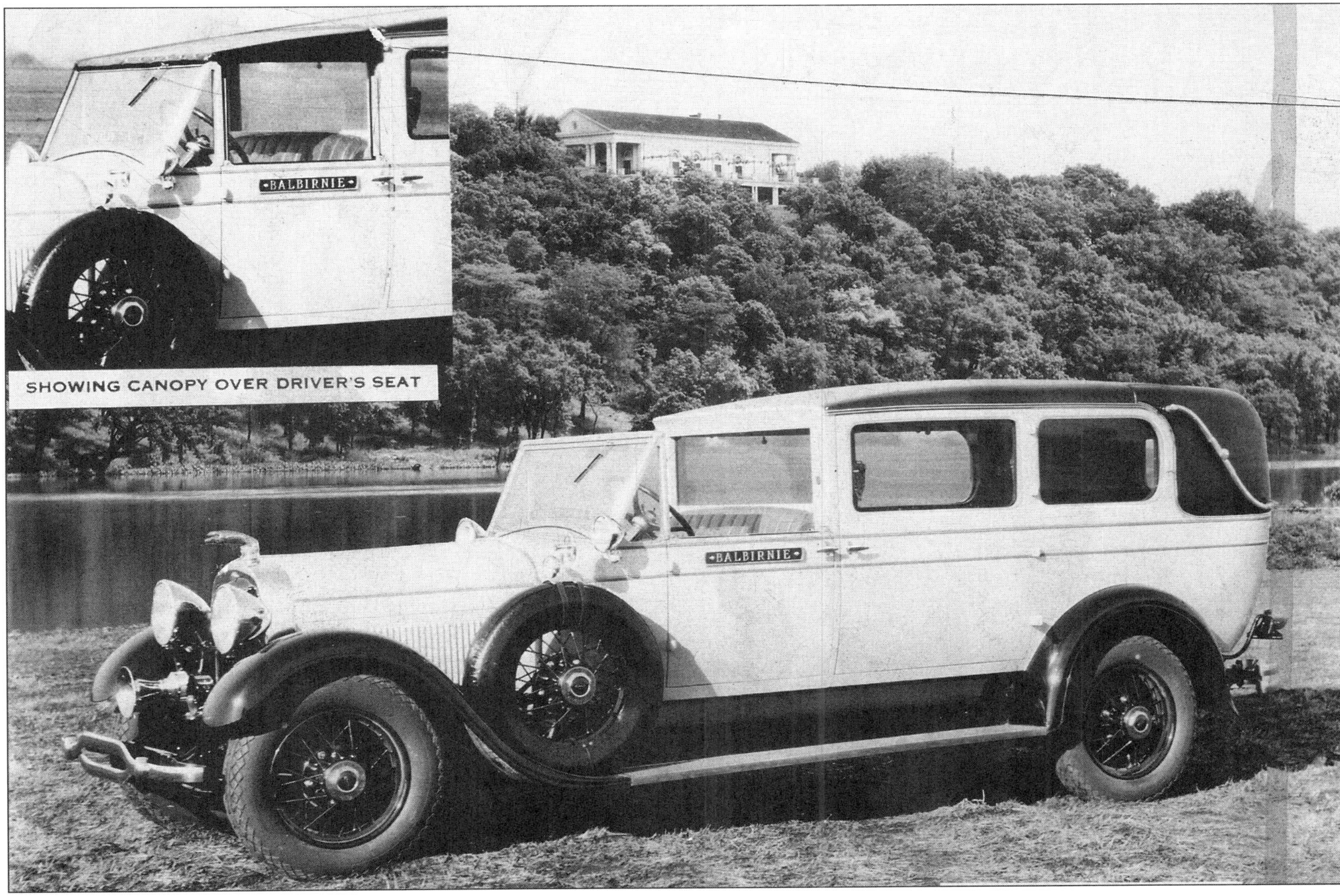

1929 EUREKA-LINCOLN TOWN CAR AMBULANCE - American ambulance design reached its zenith in the golden age of the classic car in the late 1920s and early 1930s. Just like the finest luxury cars of the day, premium ambulances had open chauffeur's compartments, padded leather-covered roofs, and eye-catching two-tone paint jobs. The Eureka Company of Rock Falls, Illinois built this Town Car Limousine Ambulance with formal "landau back" upper rear quarters on a 1929 Lincoln L-Series chassis for the Balbirnie Funeral Home of Muskegon, Michigan.

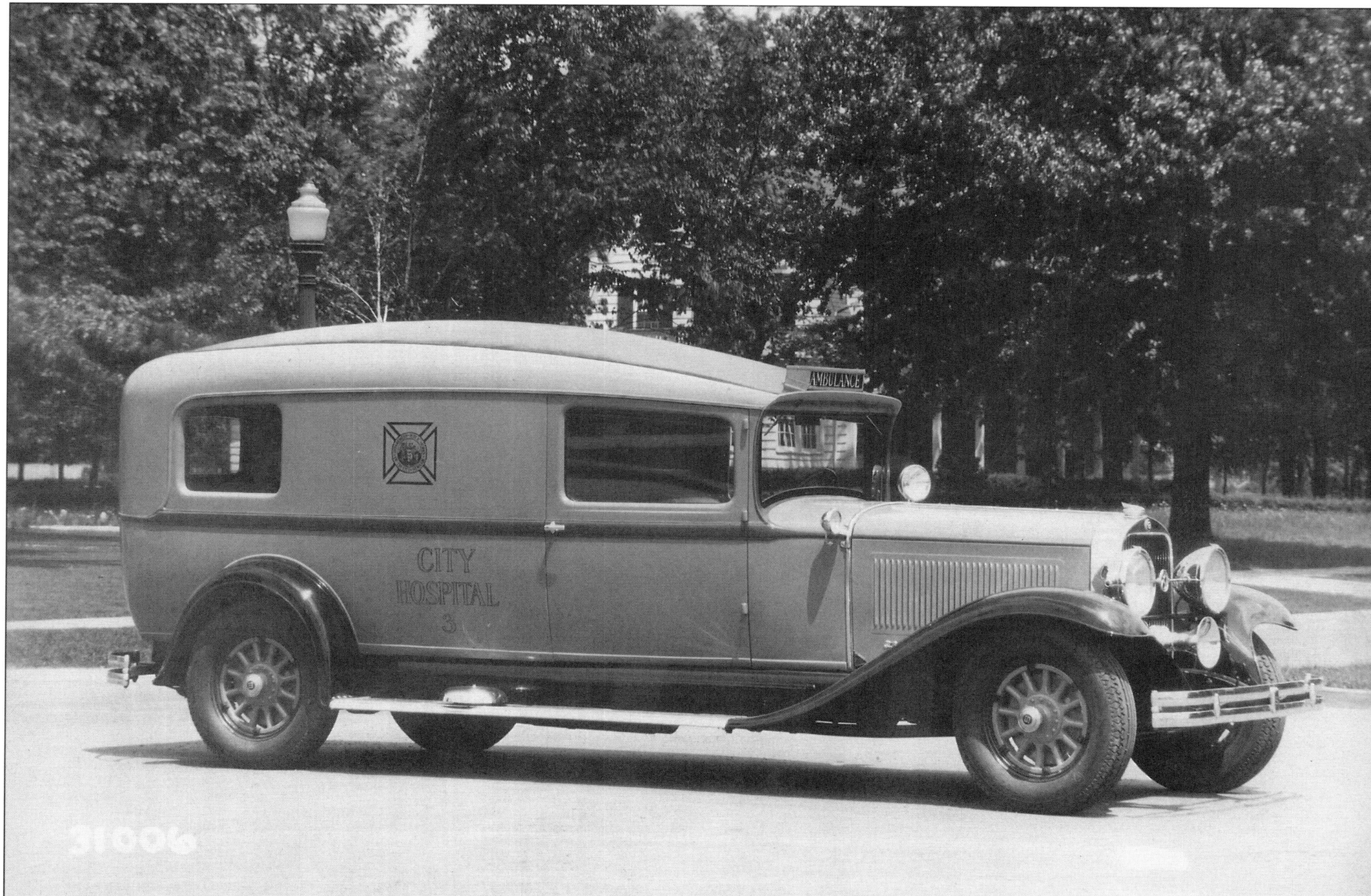

1930 SUPERIOR-STUDEBAKER MUNICIPAL AMBULANCE - The Superior Body Co. of Lima, Ohio, mounted its ambulance and funeral car bodies on Studebaker chassis almost exclusively from 1926 well into the 1930s. Superior built this special municipal-type ambulance for the City of Newark, New Jersey. Note the high, domed roofline, the gong mounted on the running board, and the illuminated “Ambulance” sign above the windshield.

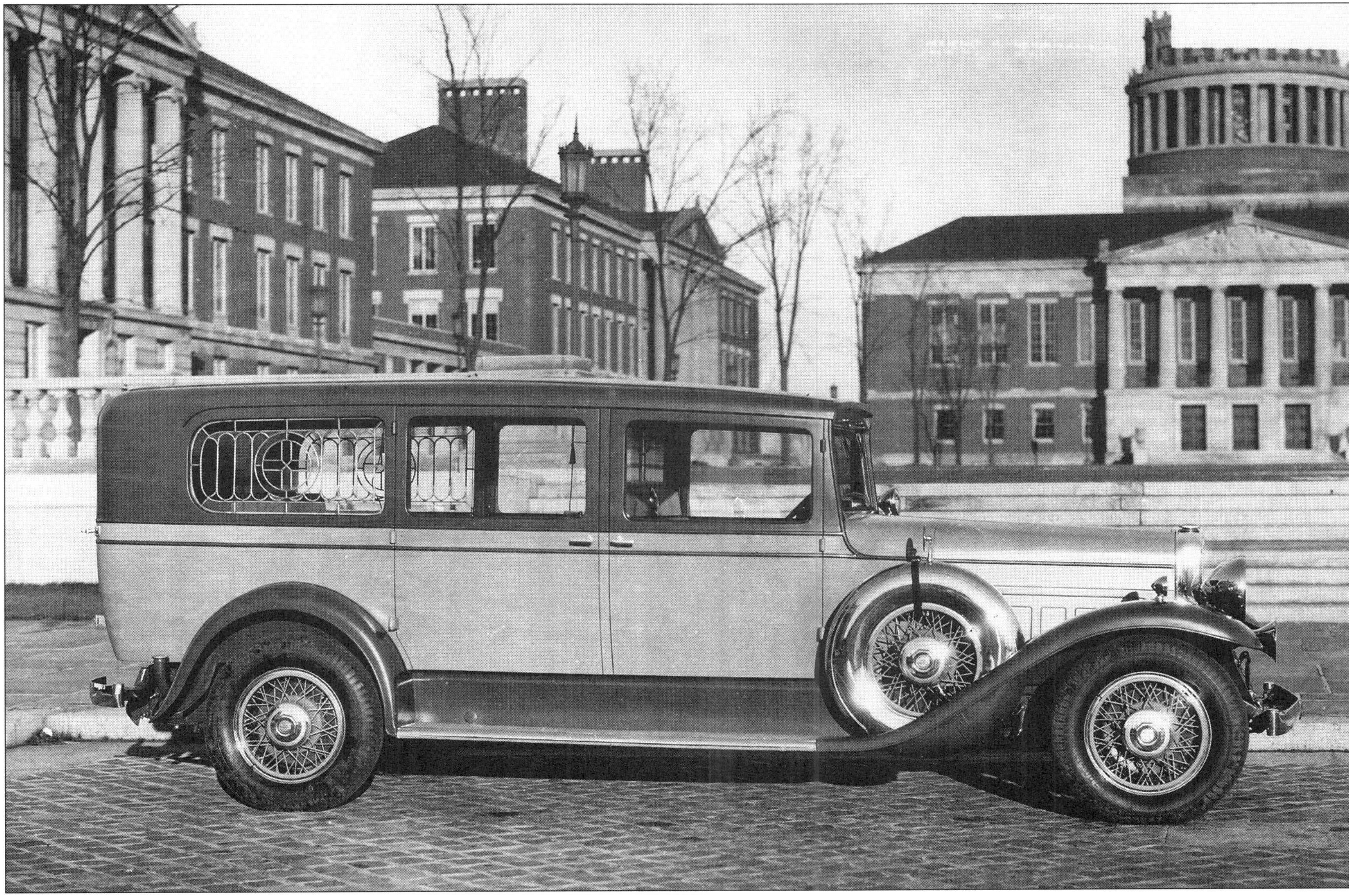

1931 CUNNINGHAM STYLE 318A AMBULANCE -The James Cunningham Son & Co. of Rochester, New York, was known for its ultra-expensive hearses and ambulances. Only the largest and most prosperous funeral firms could afford to operate Cunningham equipment. Cunningham built this handsome limousine-style ambulance with leaded rear side windows for a local hospital. Note the plated sidemount spare tire covers and wire wheels.

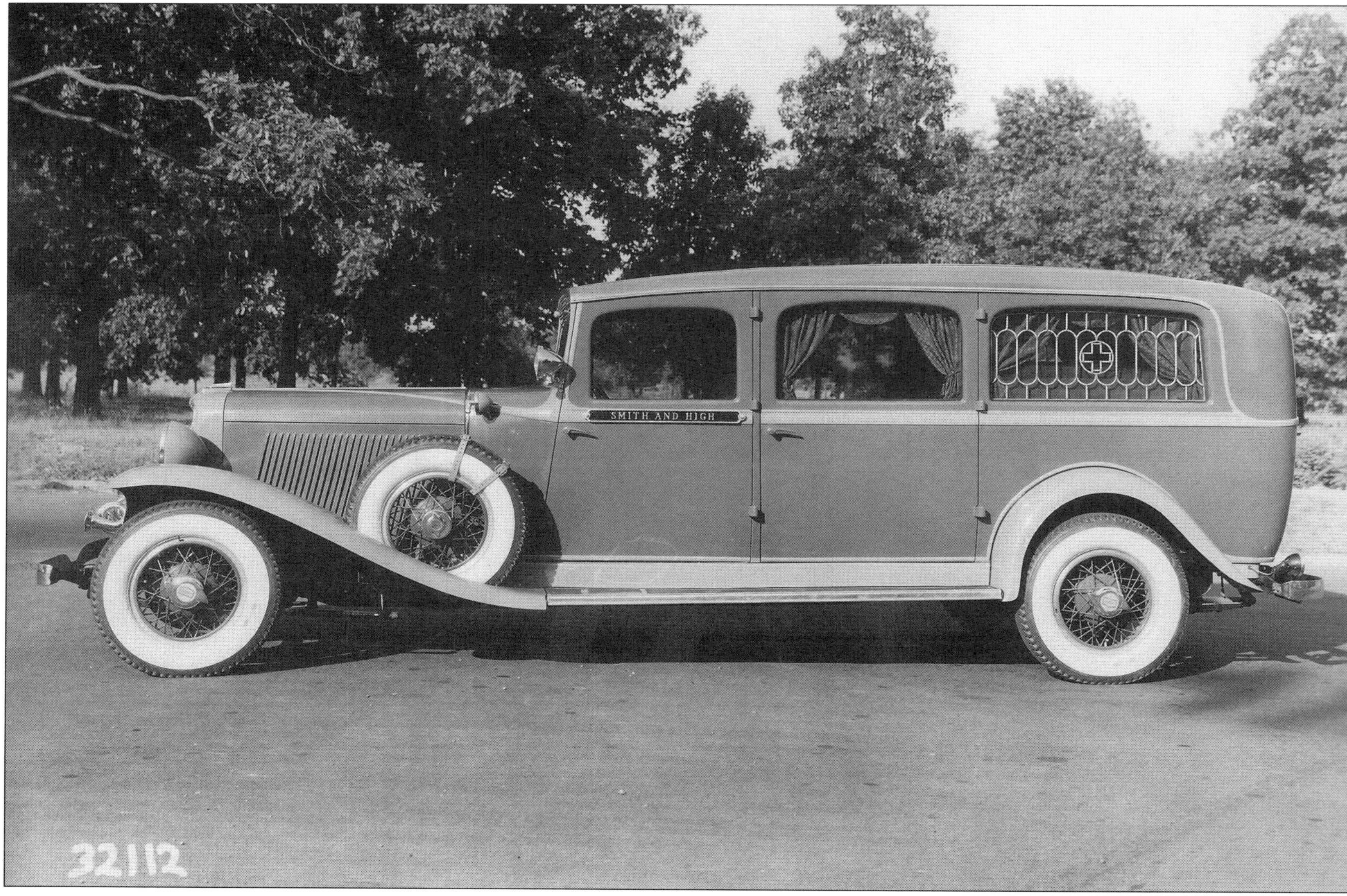

1932 SUPERIOR-AUBURN AMBULANCE - the Superior Body Co. of Lima, Ohio, built this very stylish ambulance for the funeral firm of Smith & High in 1932. Mounted on an Auburn chassis powered by a Lycoming straight-eight engine, this ambulance has rear-hinged "suicide" front doors, artistic leaded rear window glass, and heavy hearse-style window drapes. White sidewall tires give it an even more luxurious look.

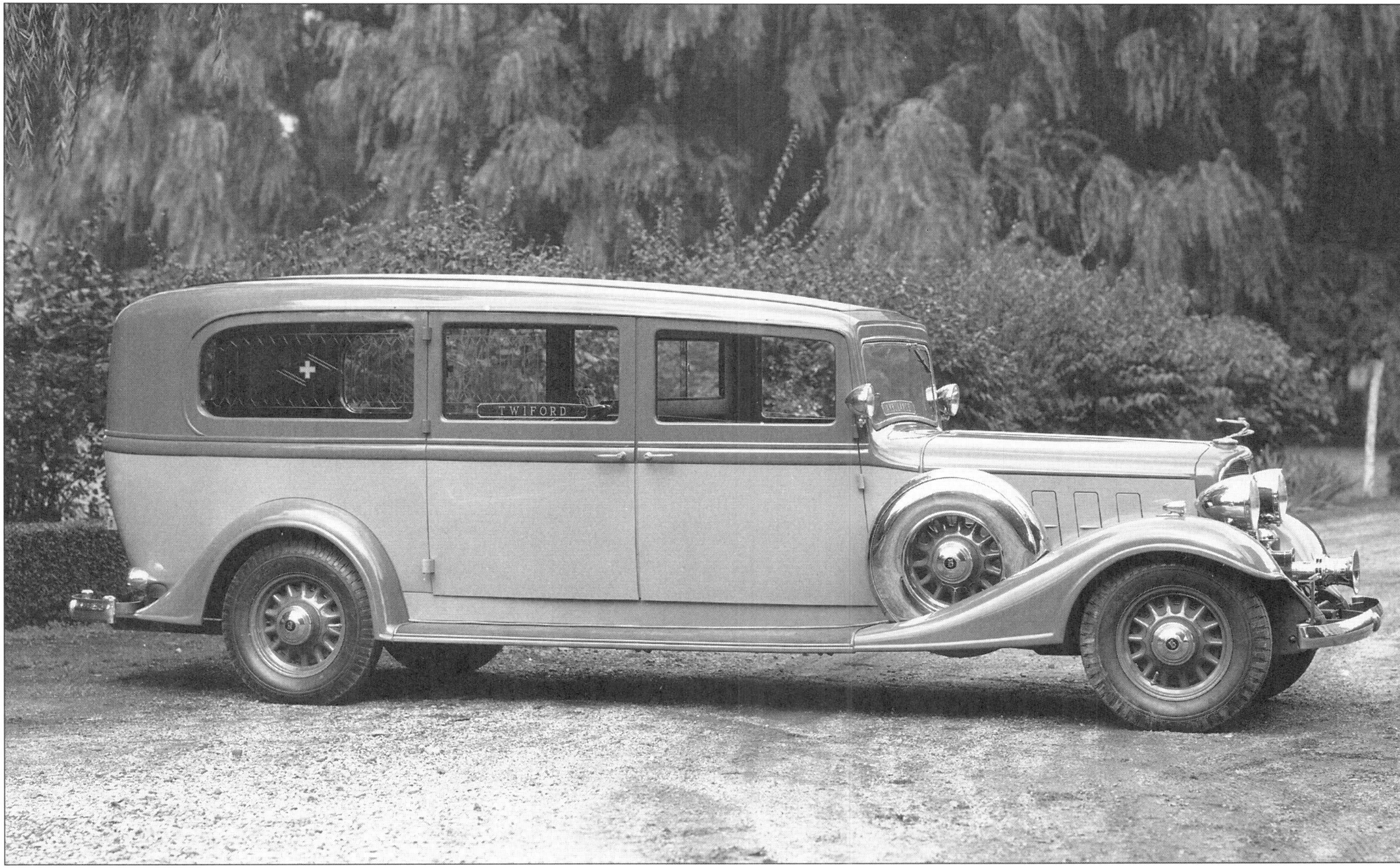

1933 FLXIBLE-BUICK PREMIER LIMOUSINE AMBULANCE - Founded as the Flexible Sidecar Co. in Mansfield, Ohio, in 1914, the company deleted the "e" in its name to sidestep trademark problems. Switching from motorcycle sidecars to buses in the early 1920s, The Flxible Co., which had relocated to Loudonville, Ohio, added hearses and ambulances to its product line in 1925. Flxible enjoyed a long and successful partnership with Buick for most of its history. Flxible built this Premier Ambulance on Buick chassis for The Twiford Co. in 1933. Note the bumper-mounted siren, dual spotlights, and chrome sidemount spare tire covers.

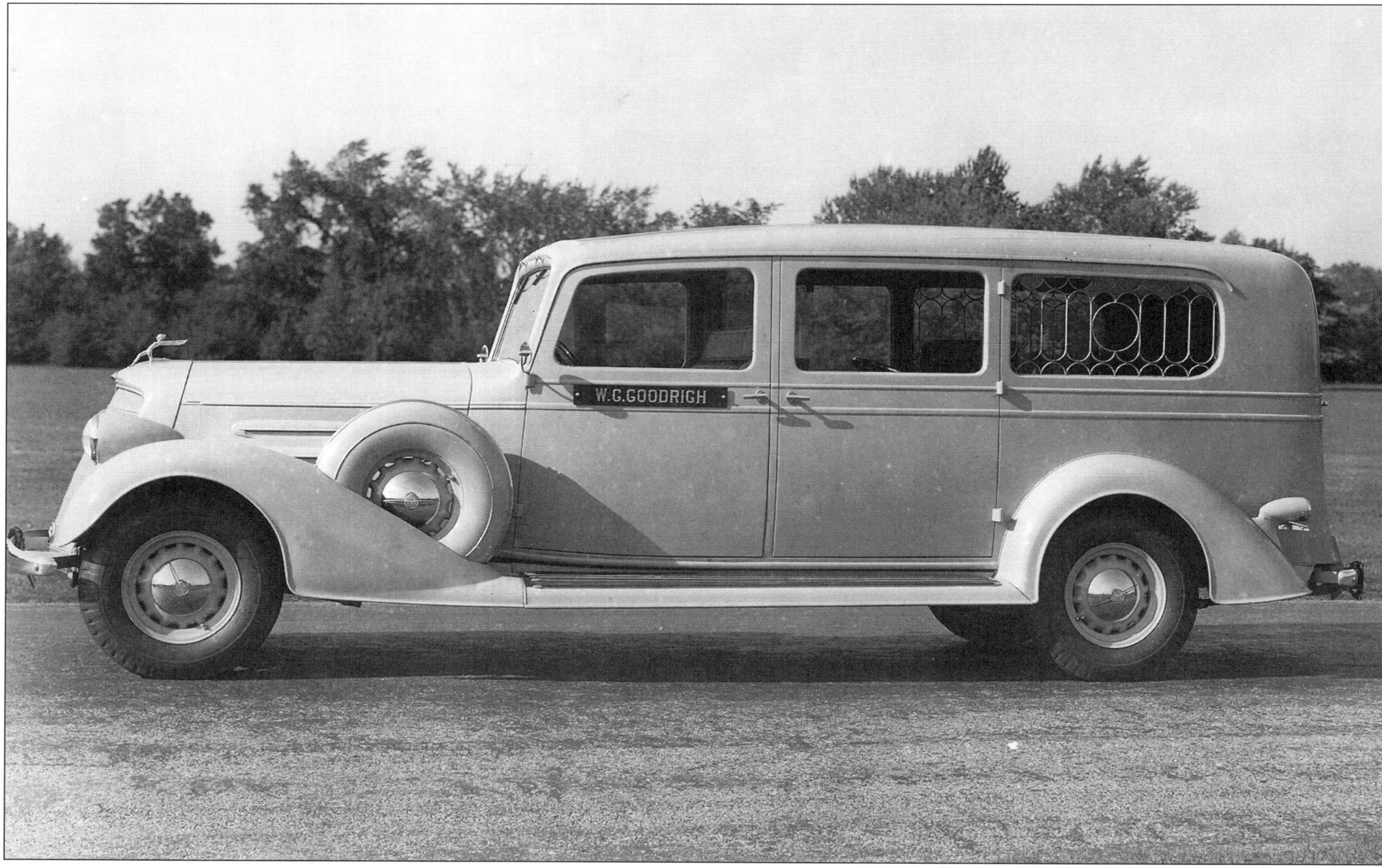

1934 CUNNINGHAM OLDSMOBILE- Faced with a precipitous plunge in orders for its luxury vehicles during the Depression, the James Cunningham Son & Co. of Rochester, New York, in a desperate bid for survival, began mounting its hearse and ambulance bodies on standard passenger car chassis. Wigan C. Goodrich took delivery of this white-painted Cunningham Limousine Ambulance mounted on the eight-cylinder Oldsmobile L-34 chassis. Not even building town car bodies for plebian Ford V-8s could save Cunningham, which ceased vehicle production in 1936, only two years before the company would have celebrated its centennial.

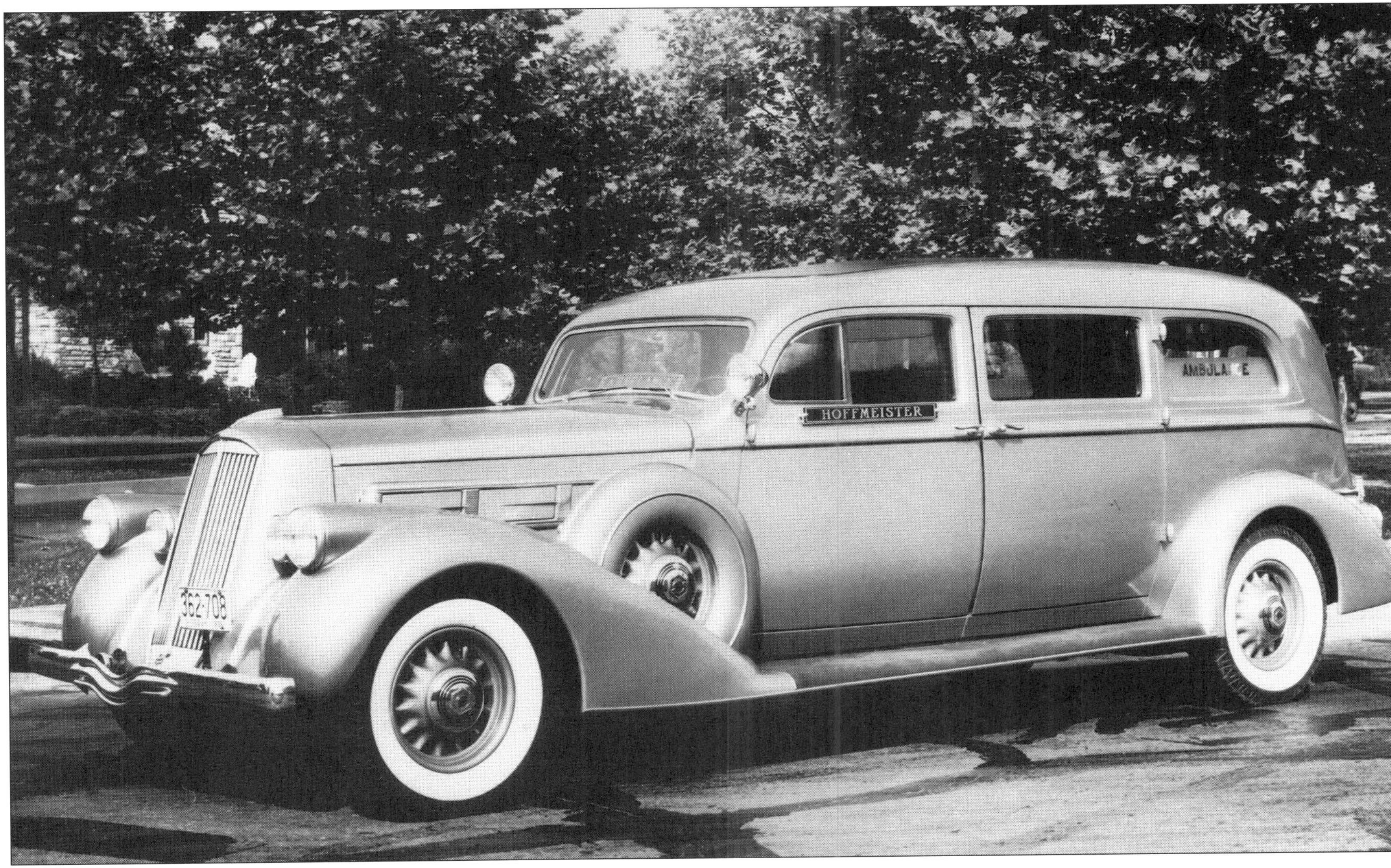

1935 HENNEY PIERCE-ARROW “ARROWLINE” AMBULANCE - The Henney Motor Company of Freeport, Illinois, is one of America’s best-remembered hearse and ambulance manufacturers. Founded in 1868, Henney was one of the largest buggy makers in the world before it entered the motor hearse and ambulance field in 1916. Henney introduced its premium “Arrowline” funeral coaches and ambulances on Pierce-Arrow chassis in 1934. The Arrowline was produced in small numbers through 1937. The Hoffmeister Mortuary of St. Louis, Missouri, was the owner of this classic 1935 Henney Arrowline Ambulance.

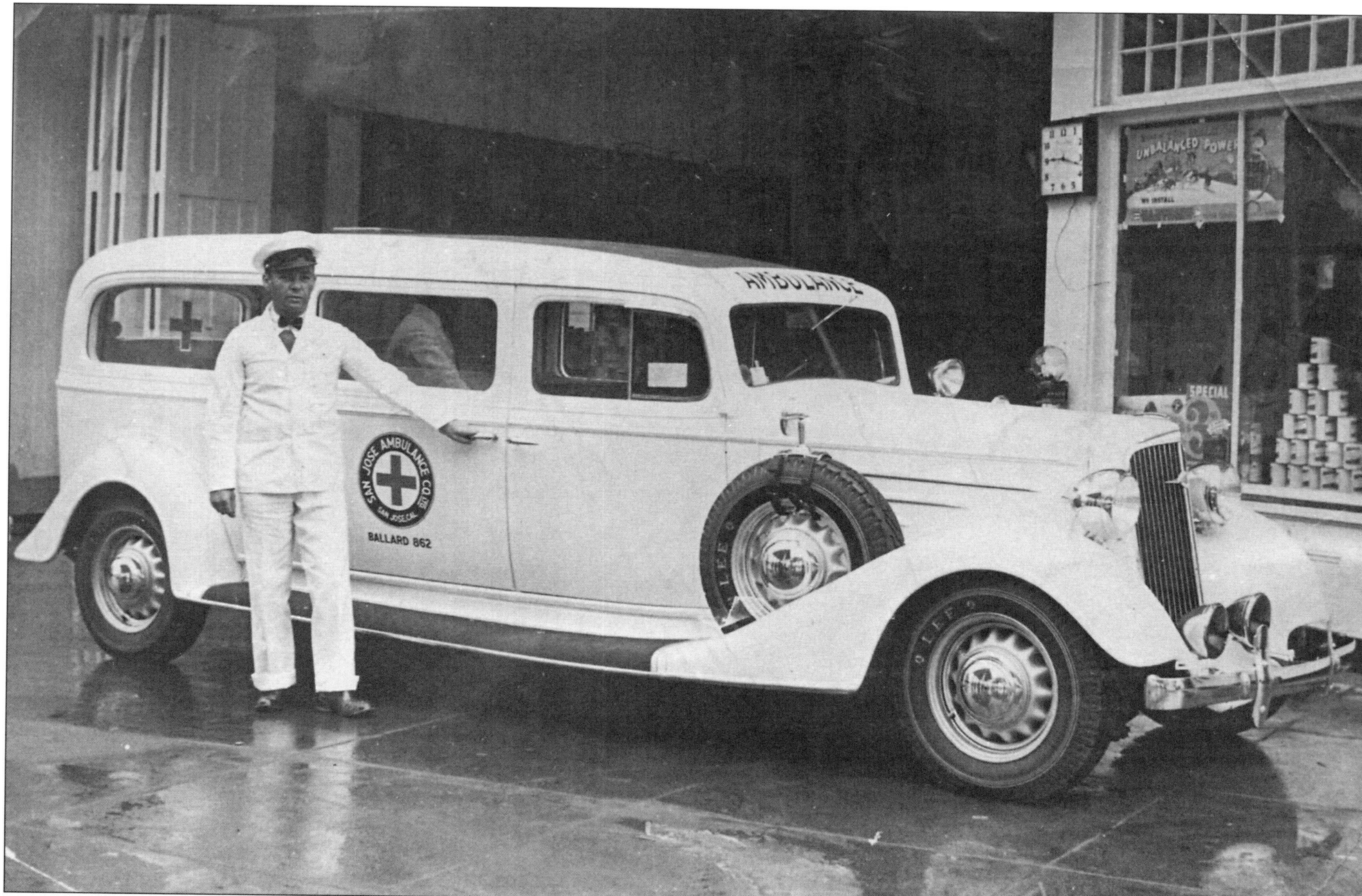

1935 CHEVROLET LIMOUSINE AMBULANCE - The builder of this 1935 Chevrolet limousine-style ambulance, which saw service in San Jose, California, is unknown. It could have been built by the Leo Gillig Works of San Francisco, or the Crown Coach Corporation of Los Angeles. The driver/attendant is attired in the standard white first aid squad uniform with white cap and black bow tie.

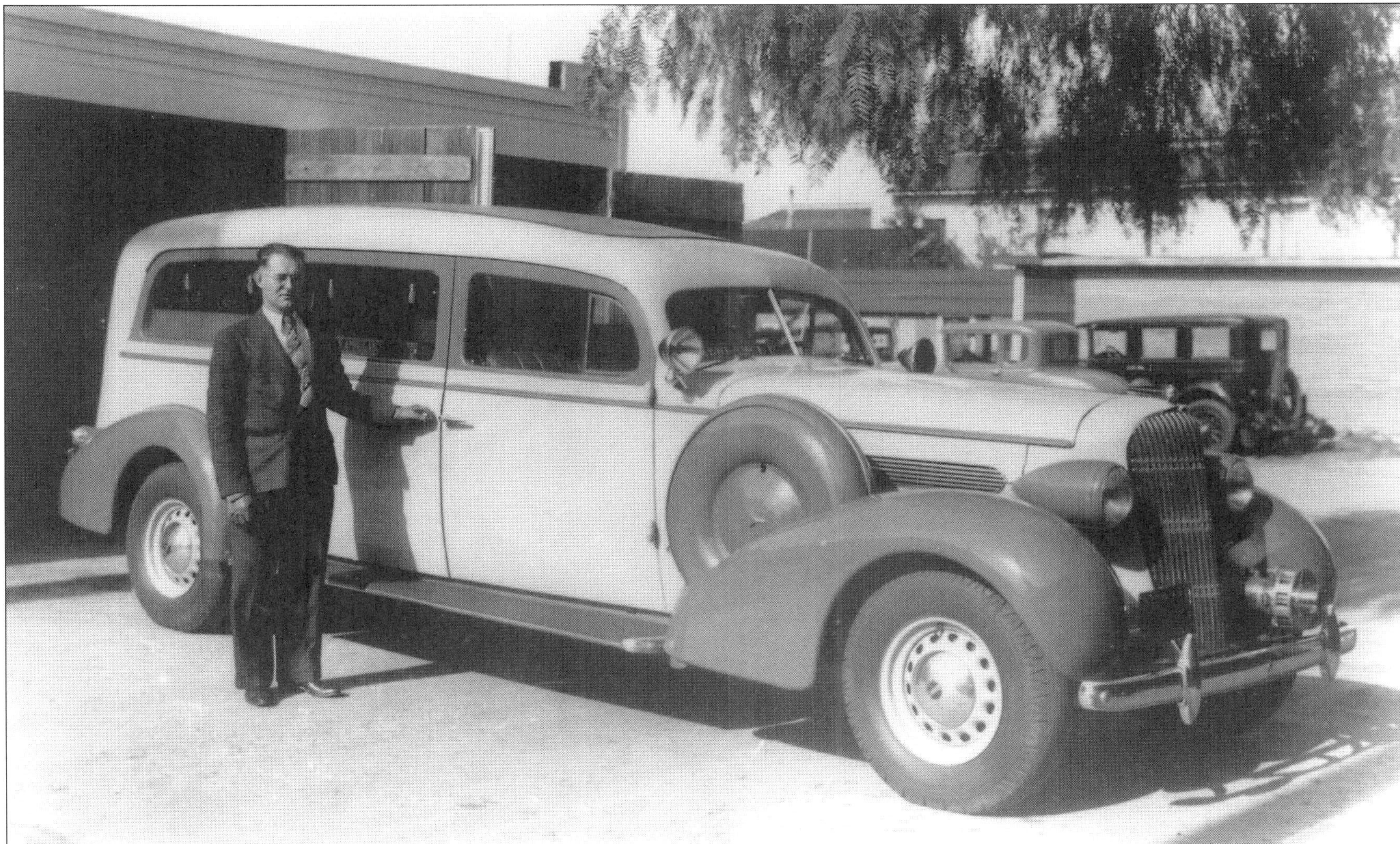

1935 HENNEY-OLDSMOBILE "PROGRESS" AMBULANCE - Faced with drastically reduced sales during the Depression, the Henney Motor Company in 1934 announced a new line of moderately priced funeral cars and ambulances built on the eight-cylinder Oldsmobile L-Series chassis. Henney's "Progress" models, available in hearse, ambulance, service car and combination funeral car/ambulance configurations, were built through the 1937 model year. The Algoe-Gundry Co. of Flint, Michigan, operated this two-tone 1935 Henney Oldsmobile Progress Ambulance.

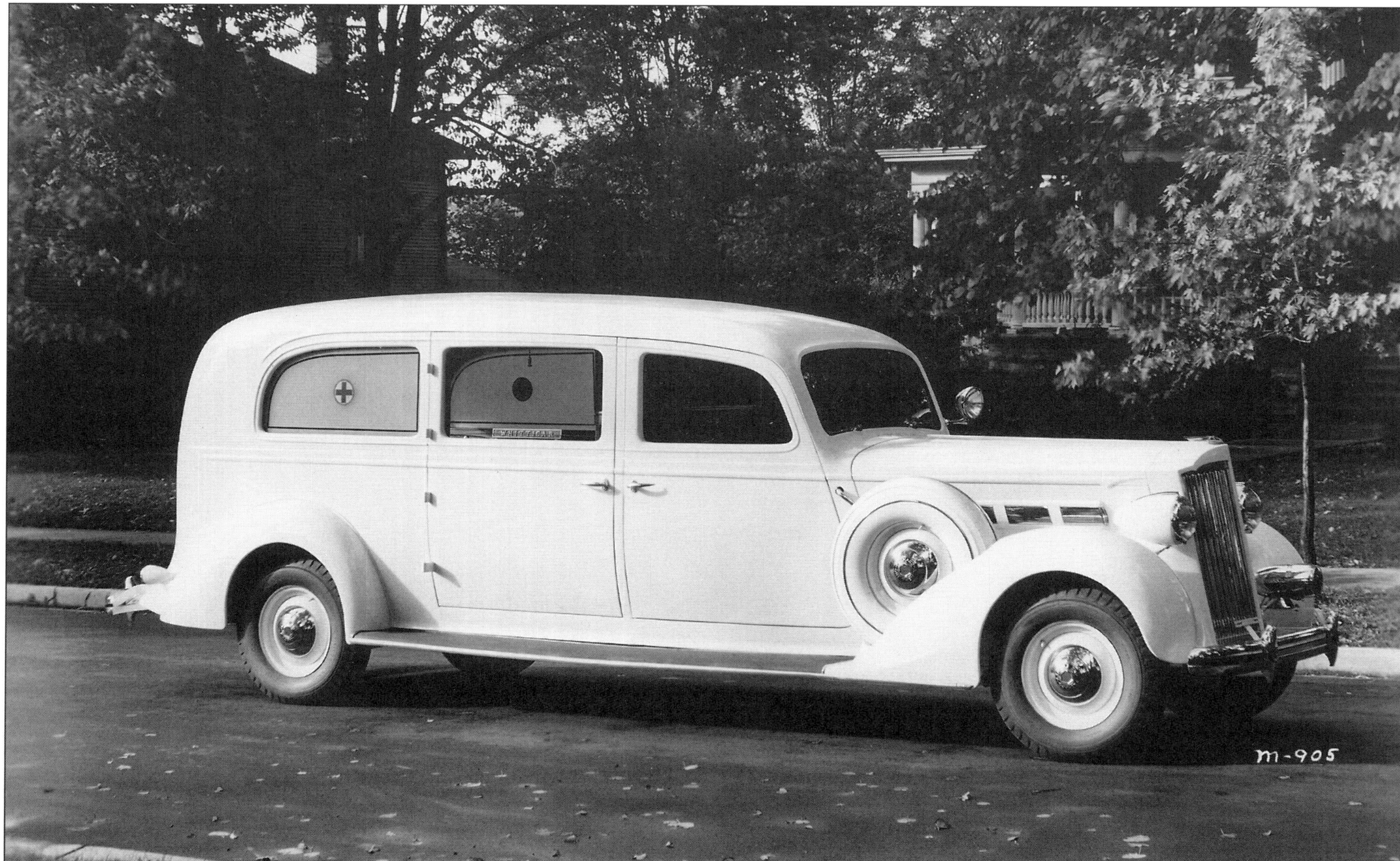

1936 MILLER-PACKARD 120 AMBULANCE - Introduced in 1935, the moderately priced Packard One-Twenty was a huge hit with America's funeral directors. In 1935, the Packard Motor Car Co. introduced a special 158-inch wheelbase "120" commercial chassis designed especially for mounting hearse and ambulance bodies. The A. J. Miller Co. of Bellefontaine, Ohio, built this Limousine Ambulance on the 1936 Packard 120-BA commercial chassis for the Whitticar Co. Note the big coaster siren mounted on the front bumper and the spotlight on the left windshield pillar.

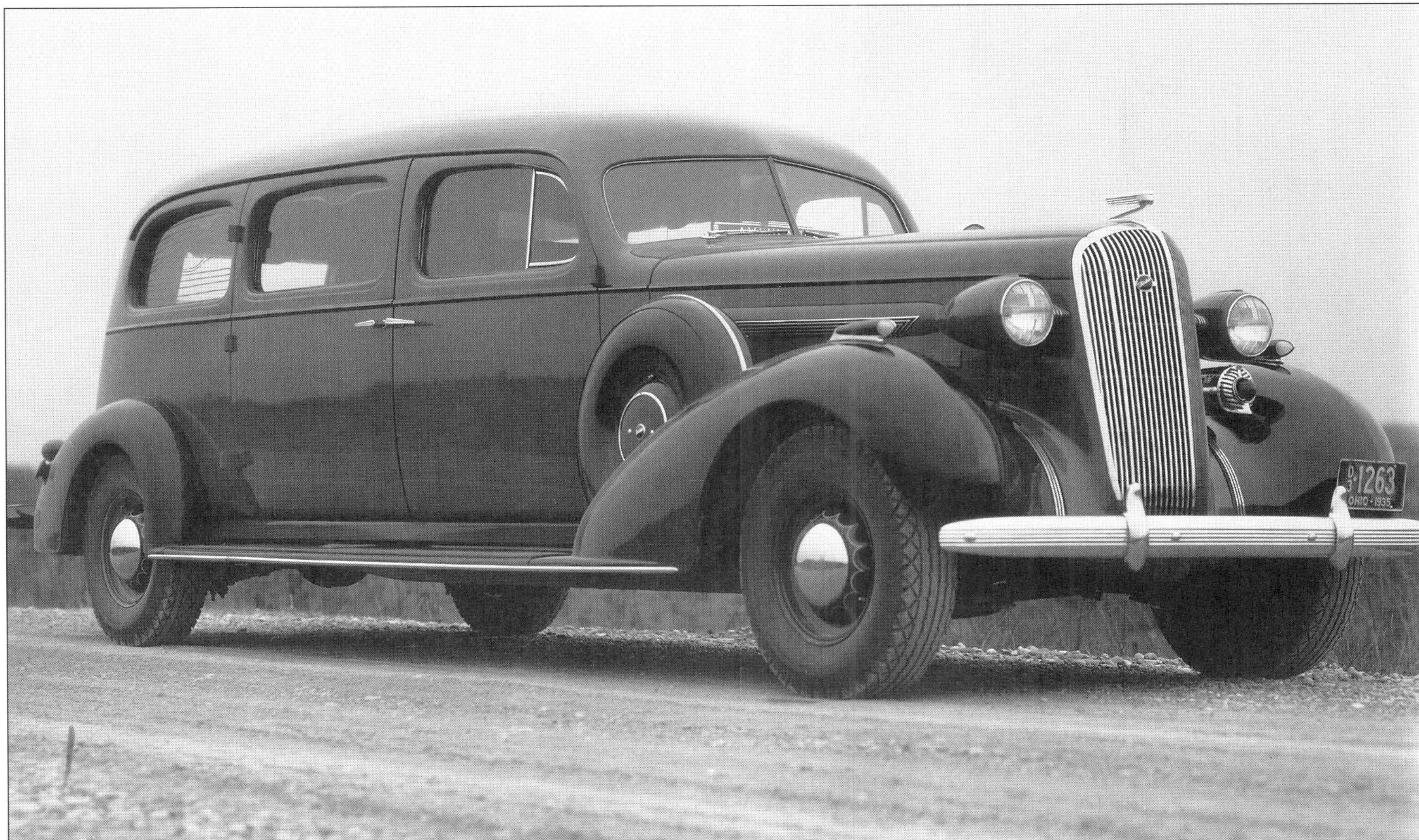

1936 FLXIBLE-BUICK COMBINATION FUNERAL COACH & AMBULANCE -For much of this century, local funeral directors provided ambulance service to their communities. While larger firms could afford single-purpose hearses and ambulances, small-town undertakers could afford only one car that had to perform dual duty as both a hearse *and* ambulance. The "Combination" was a staple product of the American funeral coach and ambulance industry into the 1970s. This 1936 Flxible-Buick is a classic Combination Funeral Car/Ambulance. Note the siren tucked under the left headlight. By the insertion of such accessories as "Ambulance" signs, attendant seats and cot locks, this car could be transformed in minutes from a stately funeral car to an ambulance.

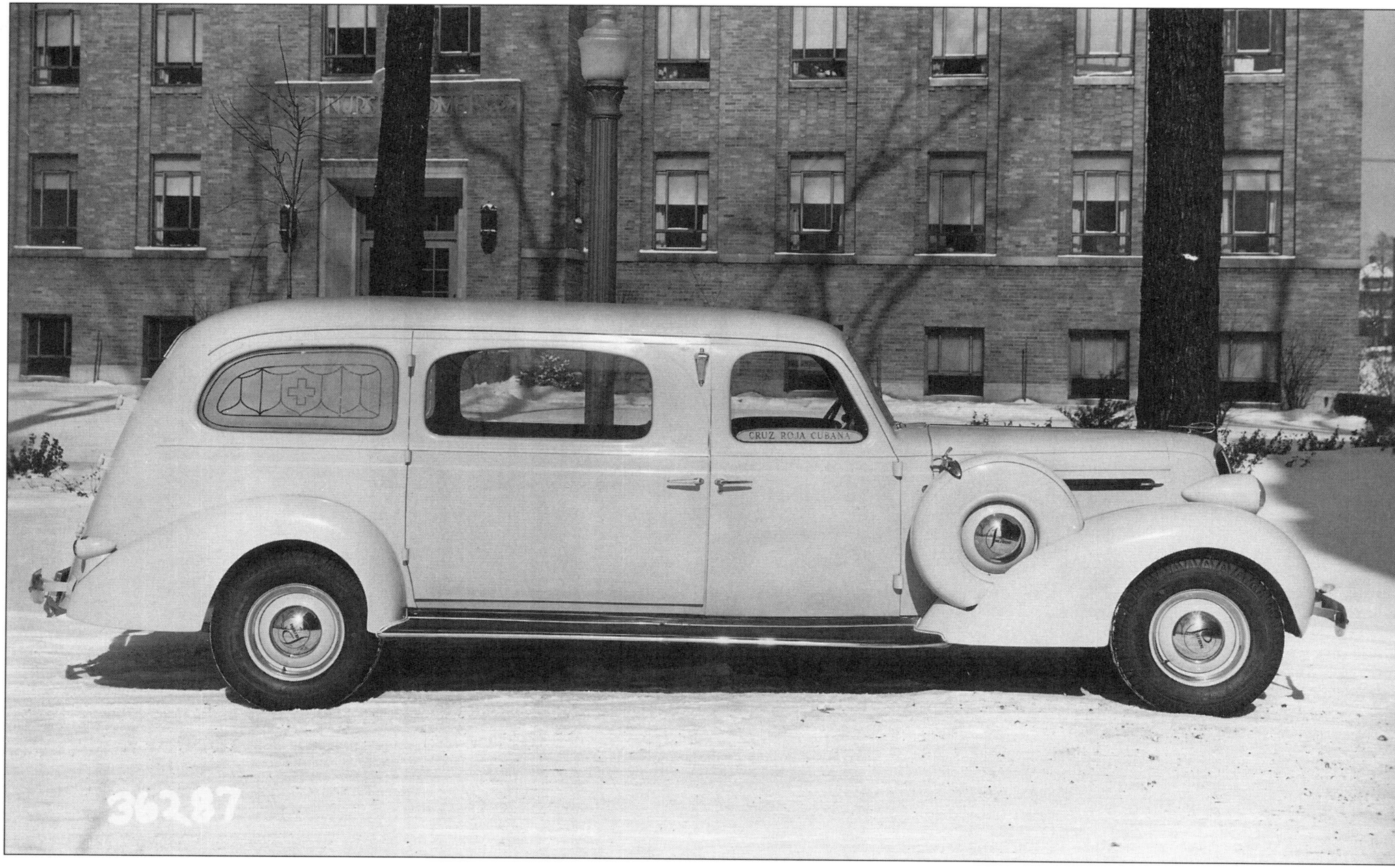

1936 SUPERIOR-STUDEBAKER "SAMARITAN" AMBULANCE - For most of its first decade in business, the Superior Body Co. enjoyed a close working relationship with Studebaker. Although the company switched to Pontiac chassis in 1936, Superior continued to market Studebaker funeral cars and ambulances through the 1937 model year. Superior delivered this gleaming white ambulance, on a 1936 Studebaker President chassis, to the Cuban Red Cross in Havana.

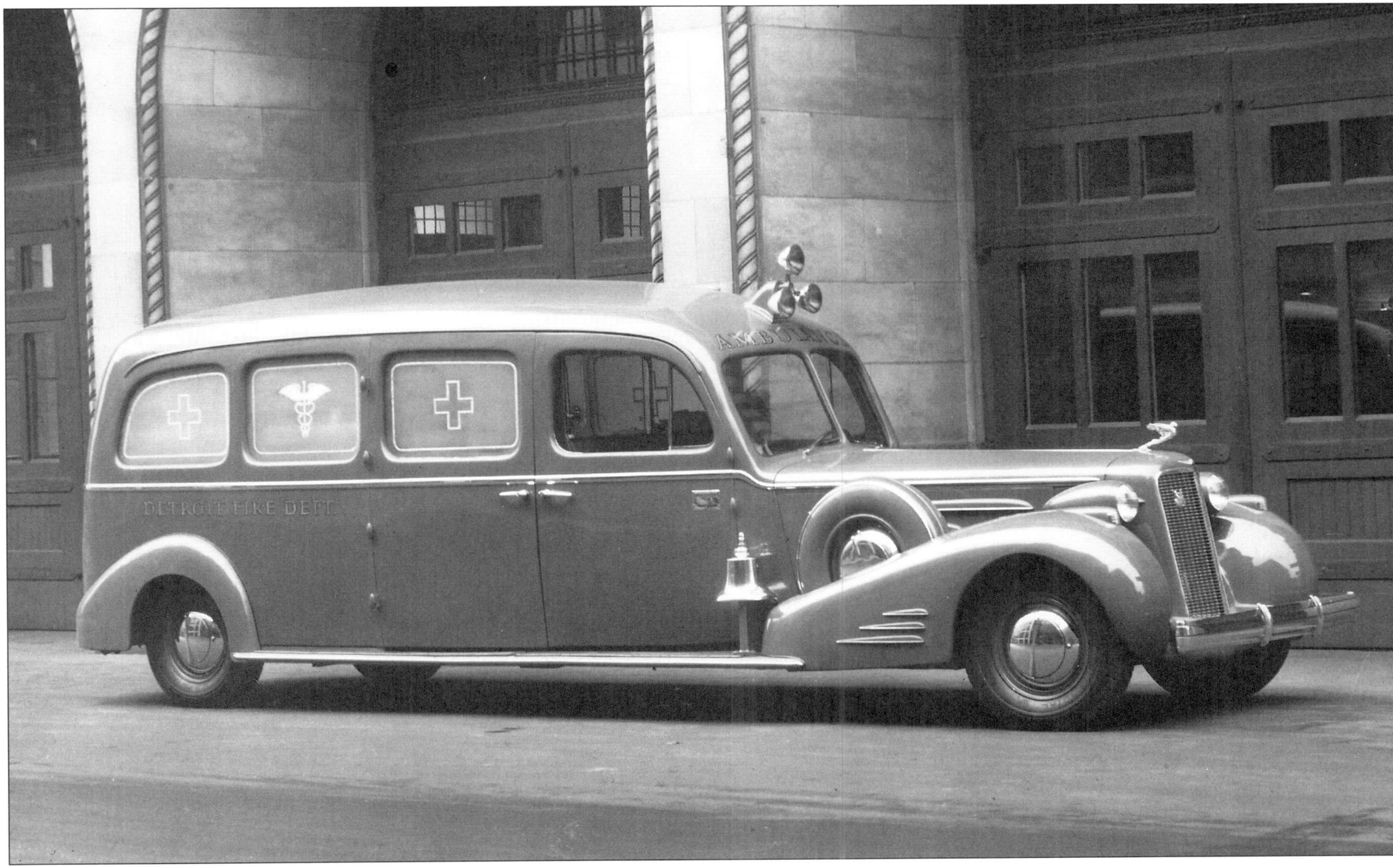

1937 METEOR-CADILLAC V-16 AMBULANCE - The Meteor Motor Car Company of Piqua, Ohio, built one of the largest and most impressive ambulances ever seen in the United States. Custom-built for the Detroit Fire Department, this one-off ambulance body was mounted on a 1937 Cadillac V-16 Series 90 chassis. A gift of Detroit Fire Commissioner Paxton Mendelssohn, the huge body was transferred to a new Cadillac V-8 chassis in 1951. The D. F. D. retired it in 1968. Note the frosted glass windows, the bell mounted behind the front fender, and the whirling Buckeye Roto-Ray warning lights above the high windshield. A true American classic!

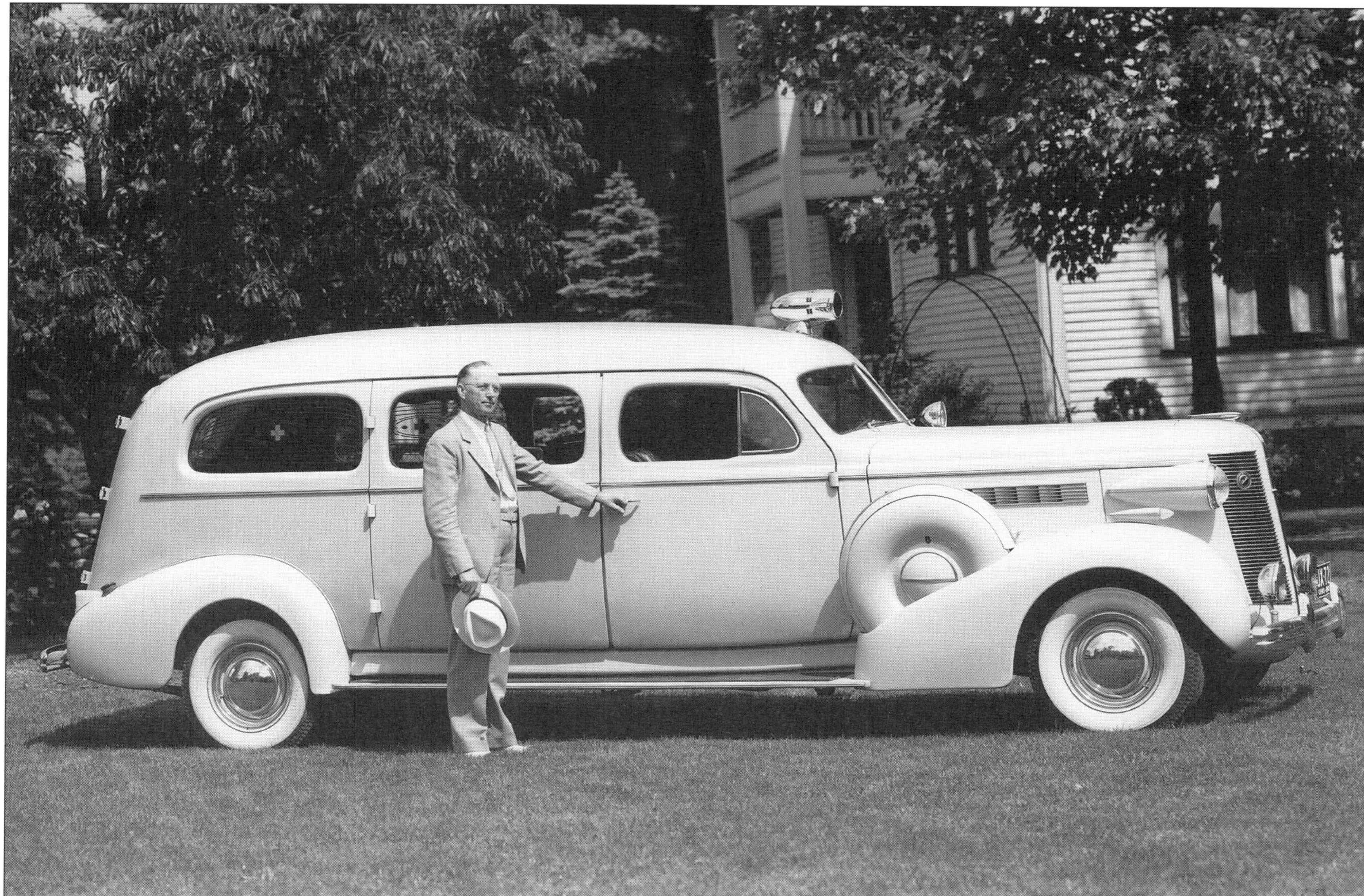

1937 FLXIBLE-BUICK AMBULANCE - A proud (unidentified) owner takes delivery of his new 1937 Flxible-Buick Ambulance at the Flxible factory in Loudonville, Ohio. The Flxible ambulance body is mounted on a 1937 Buick Special chassis. Note the dazzling white paint job, which is complemented by extra-cost white sidewall tires, and the fog lamps mounted on the front bumper.

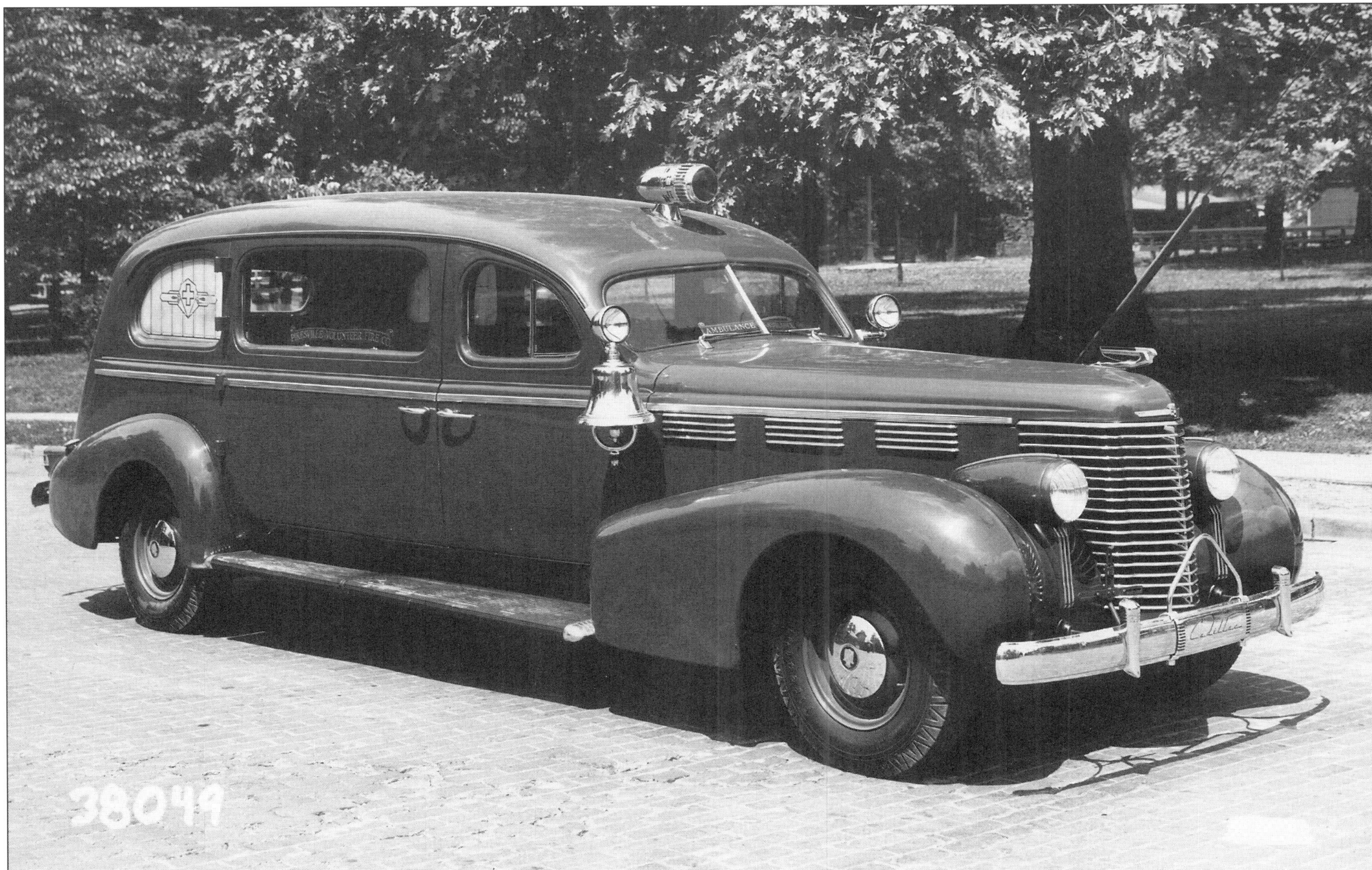

1938 SUPERIOR CADILLAC AMBULANCE - The Superior Coach Corporation of Lima, Ohio, built this impressive limousine-style ambulance on the 159-inch wheelbase Cadillac Series 60 commercial chassis for the Pikesville Volunteer Fire Company of Pikesville, Maryland. Painted Fire Department Red, it is equipped with a standard fire apparatus bell mounted on the right cowl. Note the frosted rear window glass and the front bumper grille guard. Superior listed this model as the Cambridge Ambulance.

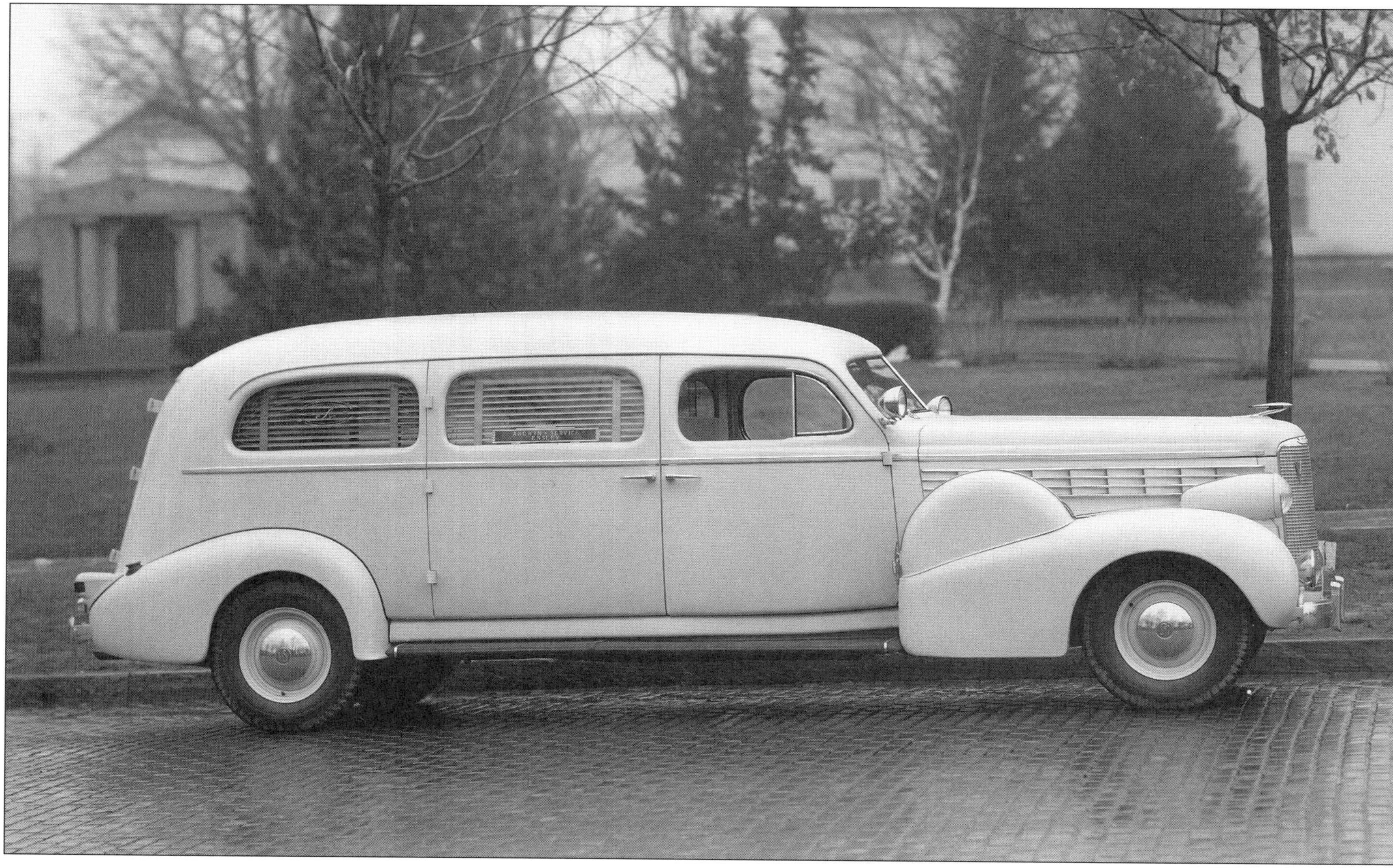

1938 FLXIBLE-LaSALLE AMBULANCE - Cadillac's sister division, LaSalle, got into the hearse and ambulance business in 1934. Like Cadillac, LaSalle offered a special long-wheelbase commercial chassis designed for hearse and ambulance bodies. The moderately priced 1938-1940 LaSalle commercial chassis was extremely popular with professional car builders. This is a Flxible limousine ambulance body mounted on the 148-inch wheelbase 1938 LaSalle Series 50 Commercial Chassis. Note the venetian blinds in the patient compartment windows of this impressive all-white ambulance.

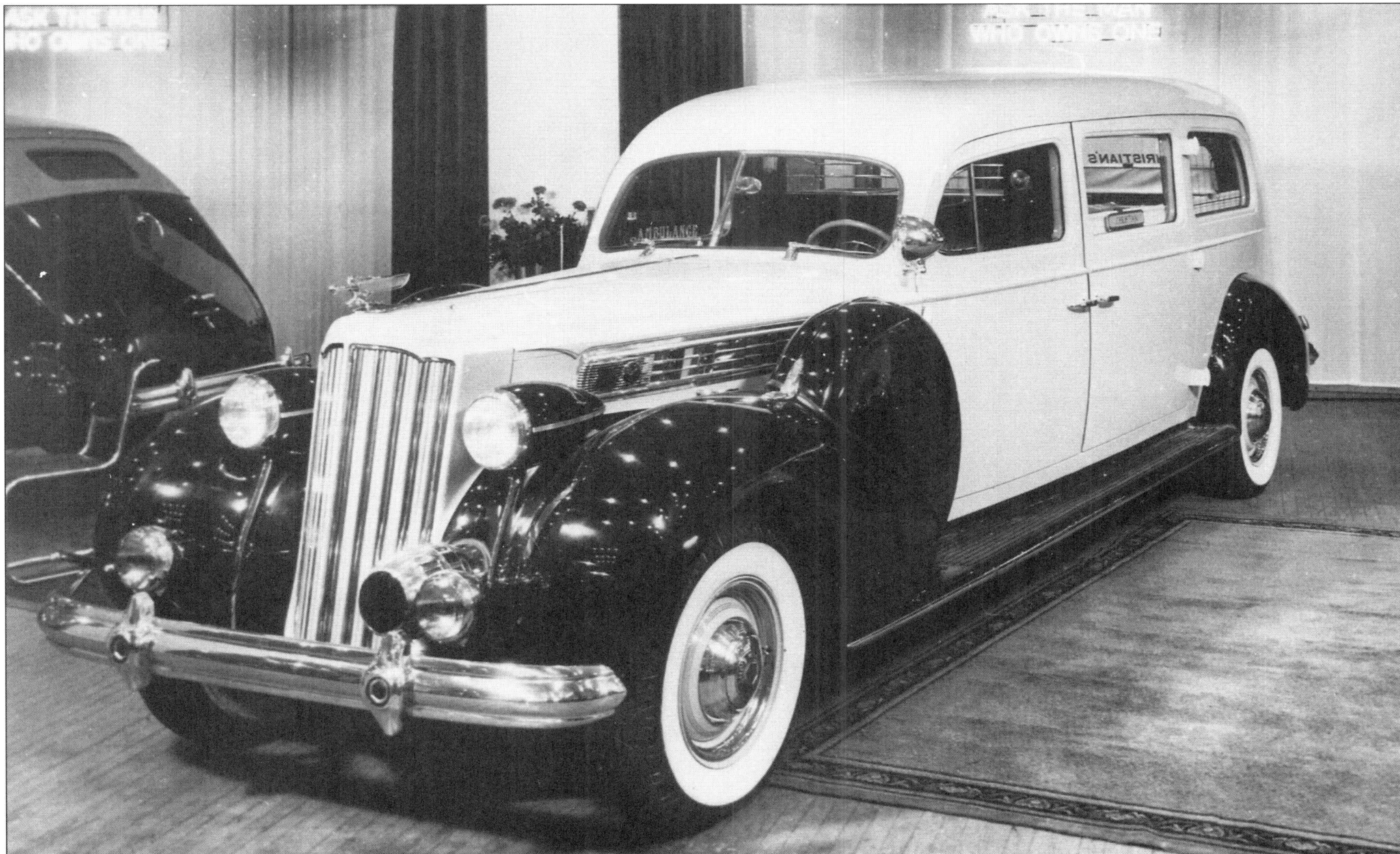

1939 HENNEY-PACKARD SUPER EIGHT AMBULANCE - In 1937, the Henney Motor Company signed an agreement with the Packard Motor Car Company under which Henney — and only Henney — could mount hearse and ambulance bodies on the Packard commercial chassis. This exclusive arrangement remained in effect until Henney's demise in 1954. This Henney-Packard Model 1594 Ambulance on the 1939 Packard Super Eight commercial chassis was photographed at the 1939 National Funeral Directors Association Convention. Henney had introduced the industry's first air-conditioned ambulance the previous year.

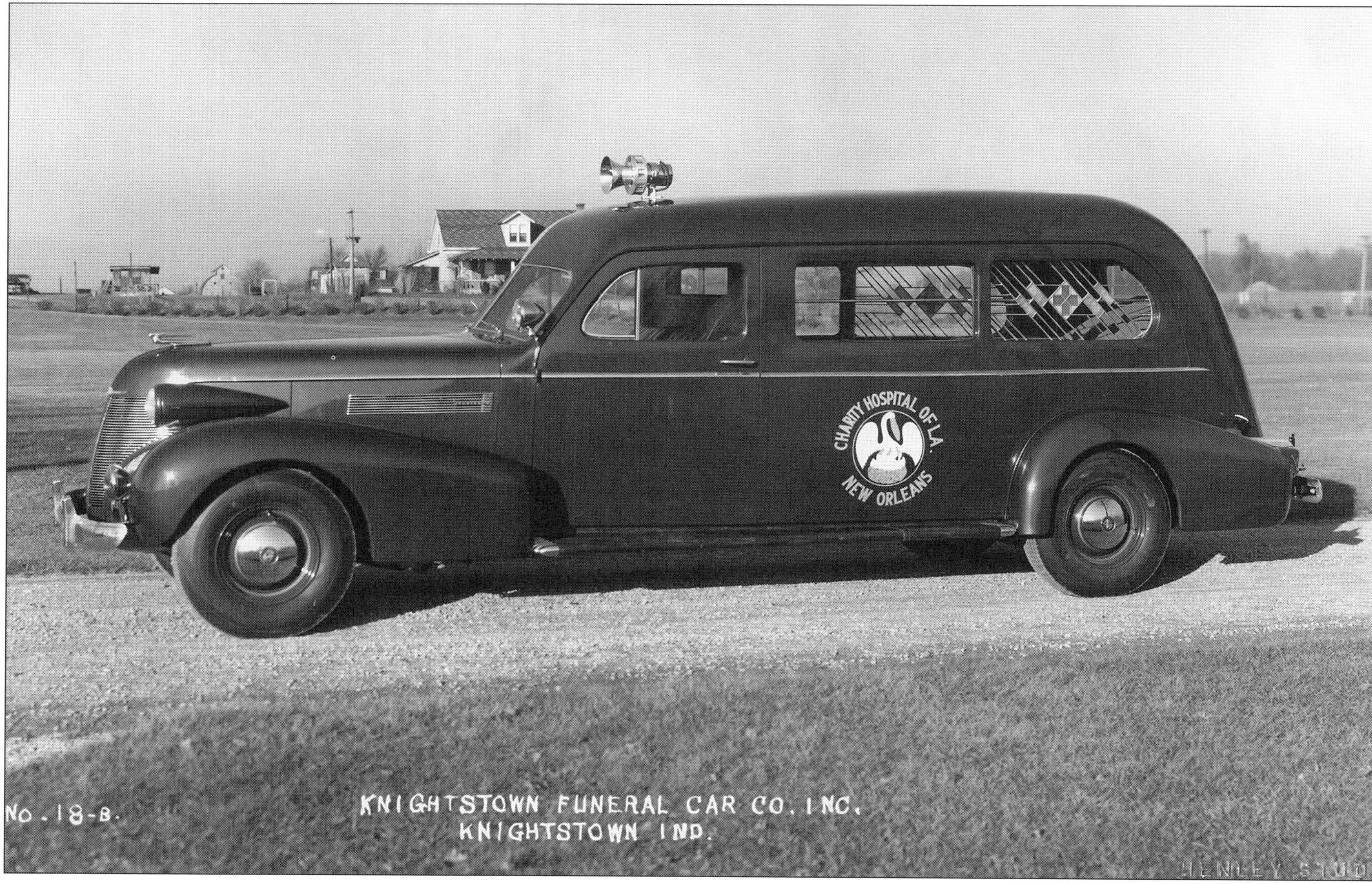

1939 KNIGHTSTOWN-CADILLAC HIGH-HEADROOM AMBULANCE - One of the smaller players in the American funeral car and ambulance industry at this time was the Knightstown Funeral Car Company of Knightstown, Indiana. This small northern Indiana town was also the home of another professional car builder, Silver-Knightstown, and later the National Body Mfg. Co. The Knightstown Funeral Car Co. built this special high-headroom ambulance on the 1939 Cadillac commercial chassis for the Charity Hospital of Louisiana in New Orleans.

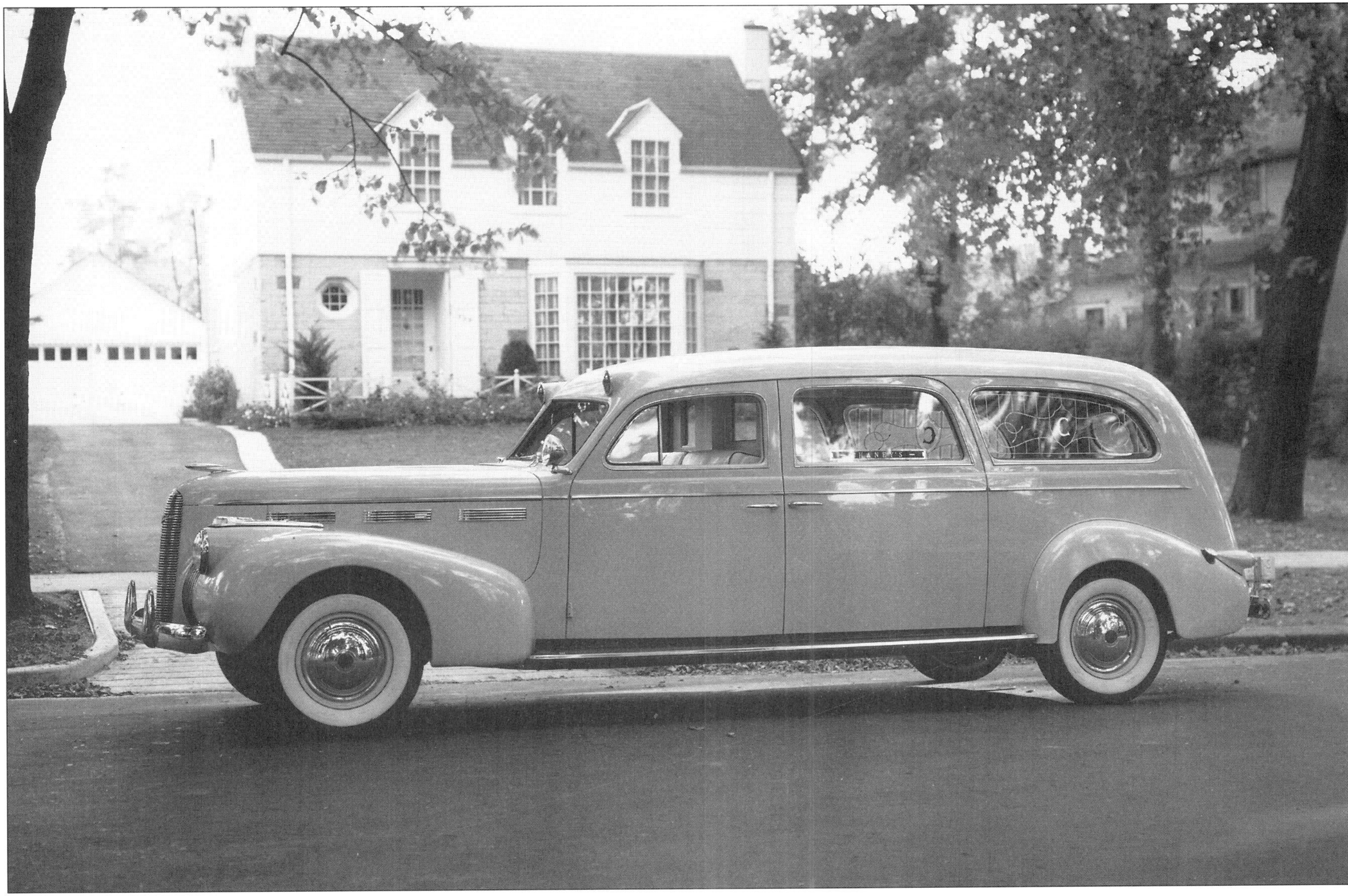

1940 MILLER-LaSALLE AMBULANCE - The A. J. Miller Co. of Bellefontaine, Ohio, built this ambulance on the 1940 LaSalle Series 50 commercial chassis. Miller's restyled 1940 bodies featured a smartly-angled "C" pillar. Note the red warning lights tunneled into the outboard edges of the roof. This would be the last year for the LaSalle. In 1941 the LaSalle commercial chassis was replaced by a new low line Cadillac Series 62.

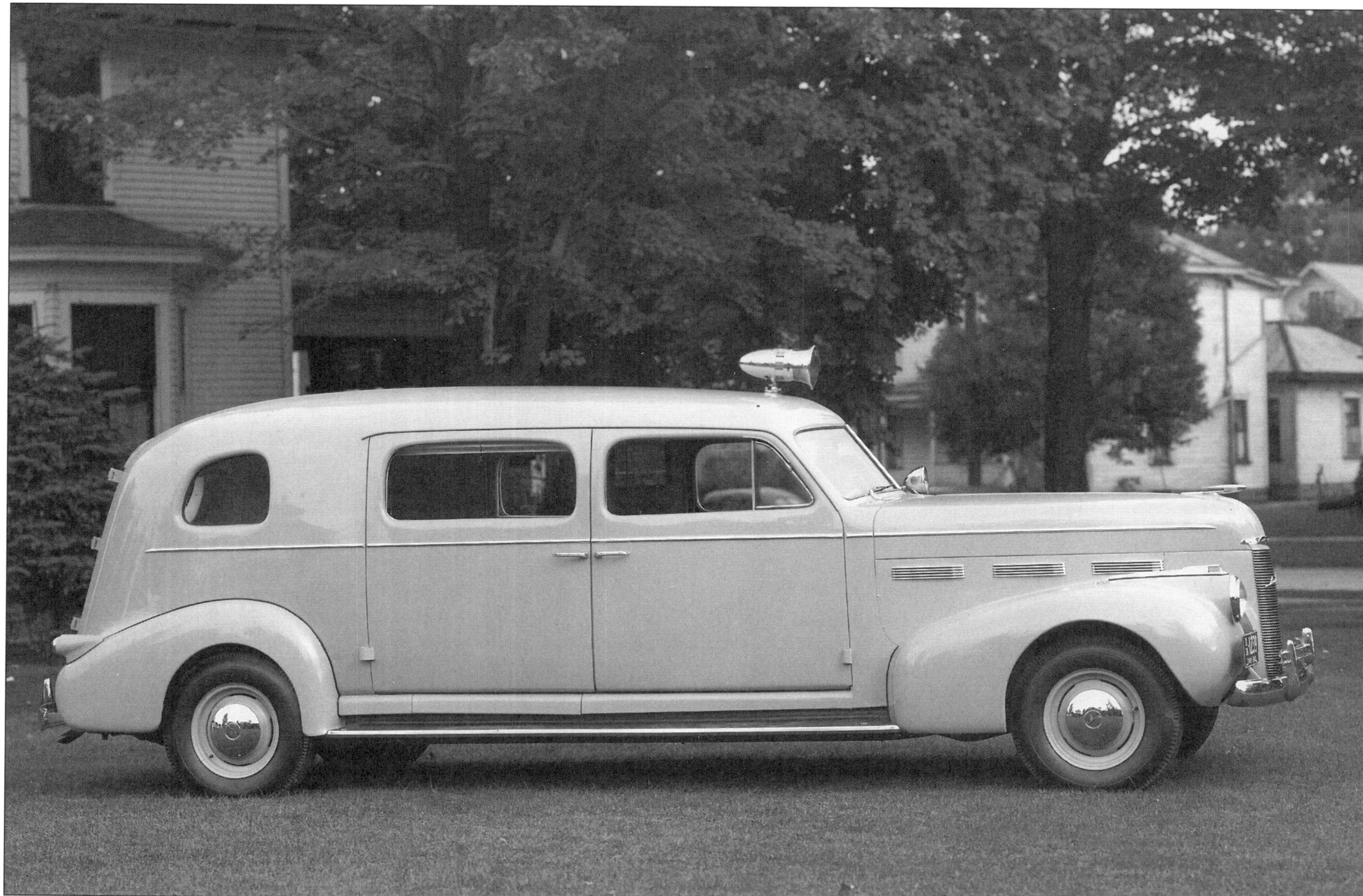

1940 FLXIBLE-LaSALLE AMBULANCE – Flxible's funeral car and ambulance bodies had unusually high beltlines, so a "fillet" was necessary to raise the base car's hood line to that of the Flxible body beltline. The built-up hood is clearly visible on this 1940 Flxible-LaSalle Ambulance. Note the unique rear window treatment; this *may* have been a military job. A roof-mounted Sterling Model 30 SirenLite clears the way.

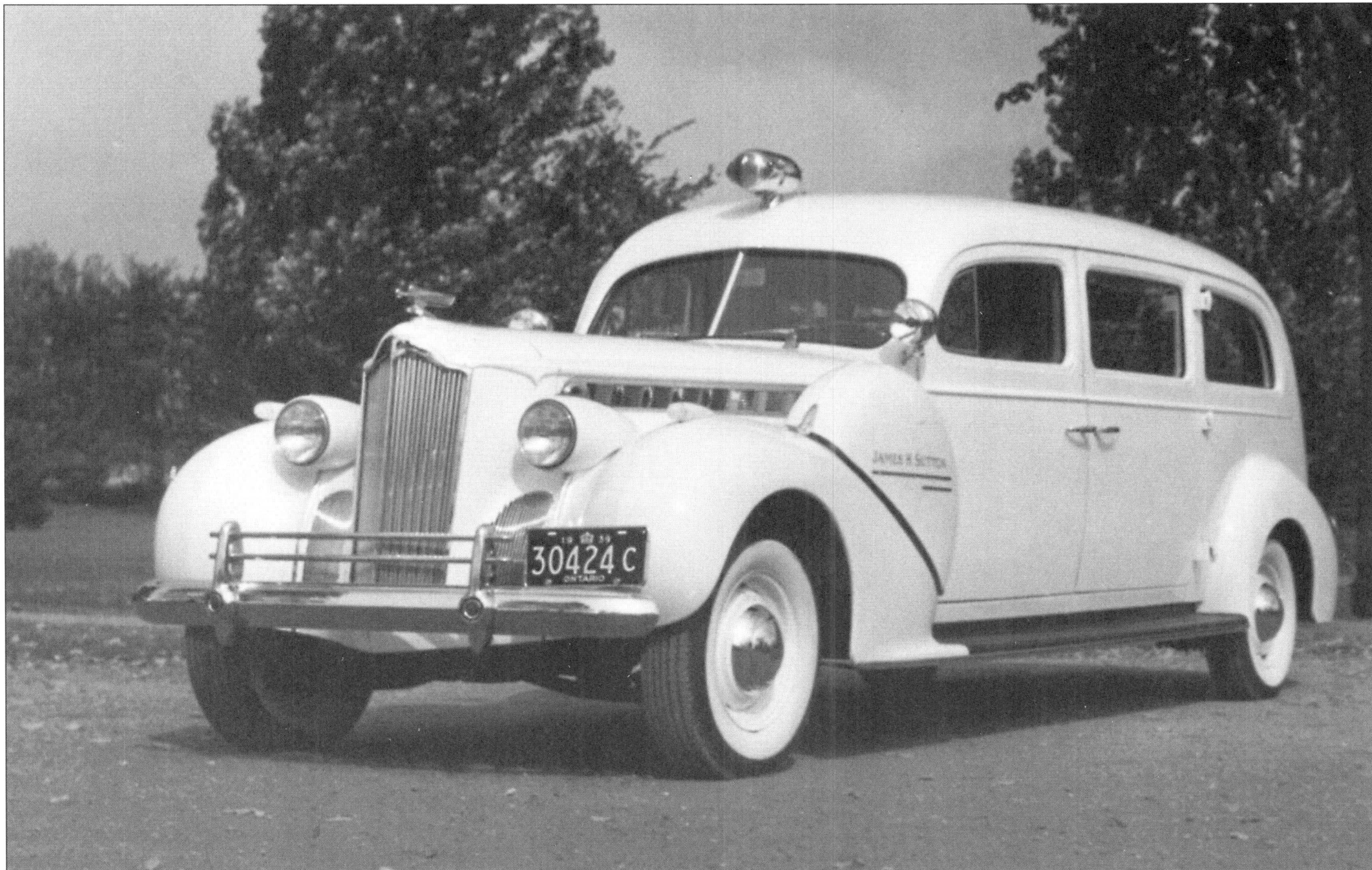

1940 BRANTFORD HENNEY-PACKARD AMBULANCE - In 1935 the Brantford Coach & Body Co. of Brantford, Ontario, entered into an agreement with the Henney Motor Co. under which Brantford was licensed to build and sell Henney-bodied funeral cars and ambulances in Canada. Brantford Coach & Body Co. sold this attractive white 1940 Brantford Henney-Packard Ambulance to the James H. Sutton Funeral Home in Windsor, Ontario. Note the grille guard and roof-mounted siren.

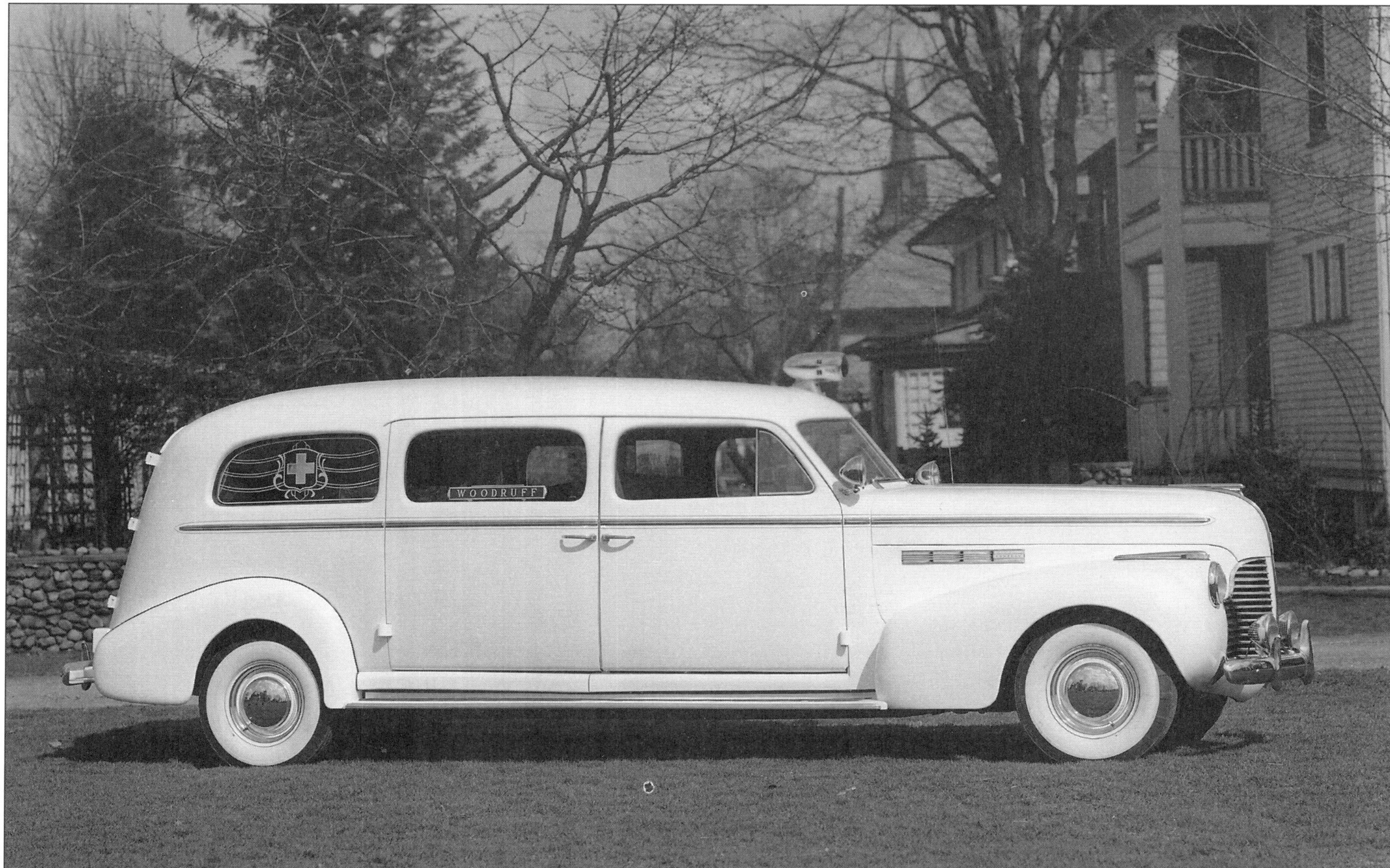

1940 FLXIBLE-BUICK AMBULANCE - The Flxible Company built this good-looking straight ambulance for The Woodruff Co. Note the ambulance cross design in the rear quarter windows, the roof-mounted siren, and the wide white sidewall tires. Unlike Cadillac and Packard, Buick did not offer a long-wheelbase commercial chassis for hearse and ambulance builders. Flxible spliced and stretched the Buick chassis/cowl units drop-shipped at the Loudonville, Ohio, plant.

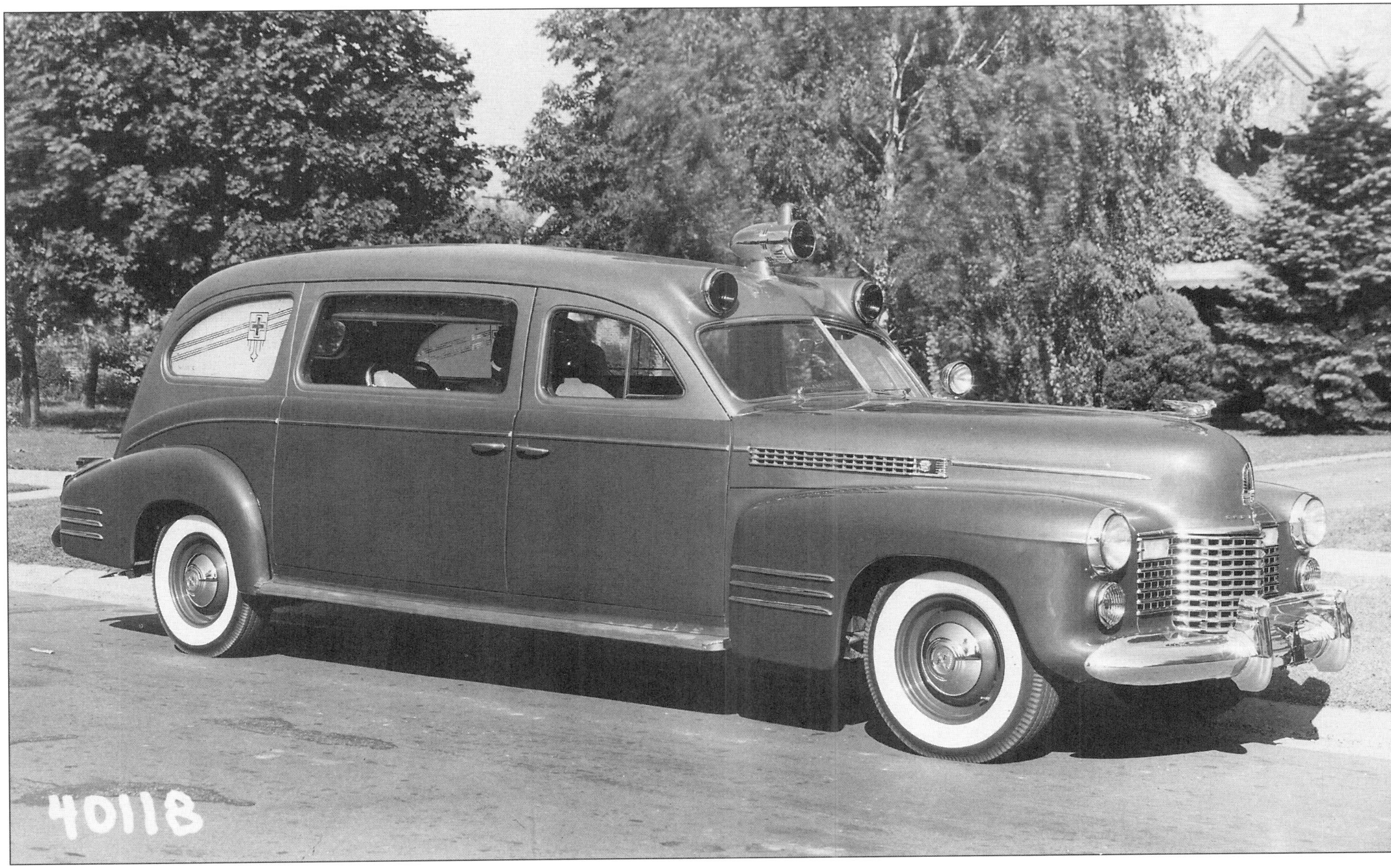

1941 SUPERIOR-CADILLAC DEVONSHIRE AMBULANCE - The 1941 Cadillac is arguably one of the best looking cars in the Cadillac Motor Division's long history. The same goes for 1941 Cadillac-chassised professional cars. The Superior Coach Corp. restyled its hearse and ambulance bodies in 1939. The new look included huge, 55-inch wide rear side doors and a body character line that swept gracefully down to the rear of the car. This is the 1941 Superior-Cadillac Devonshire Ambulance built on the new Series 62 commercial chassis. Note the tunnel roof lights and Federal Traffic King siren.

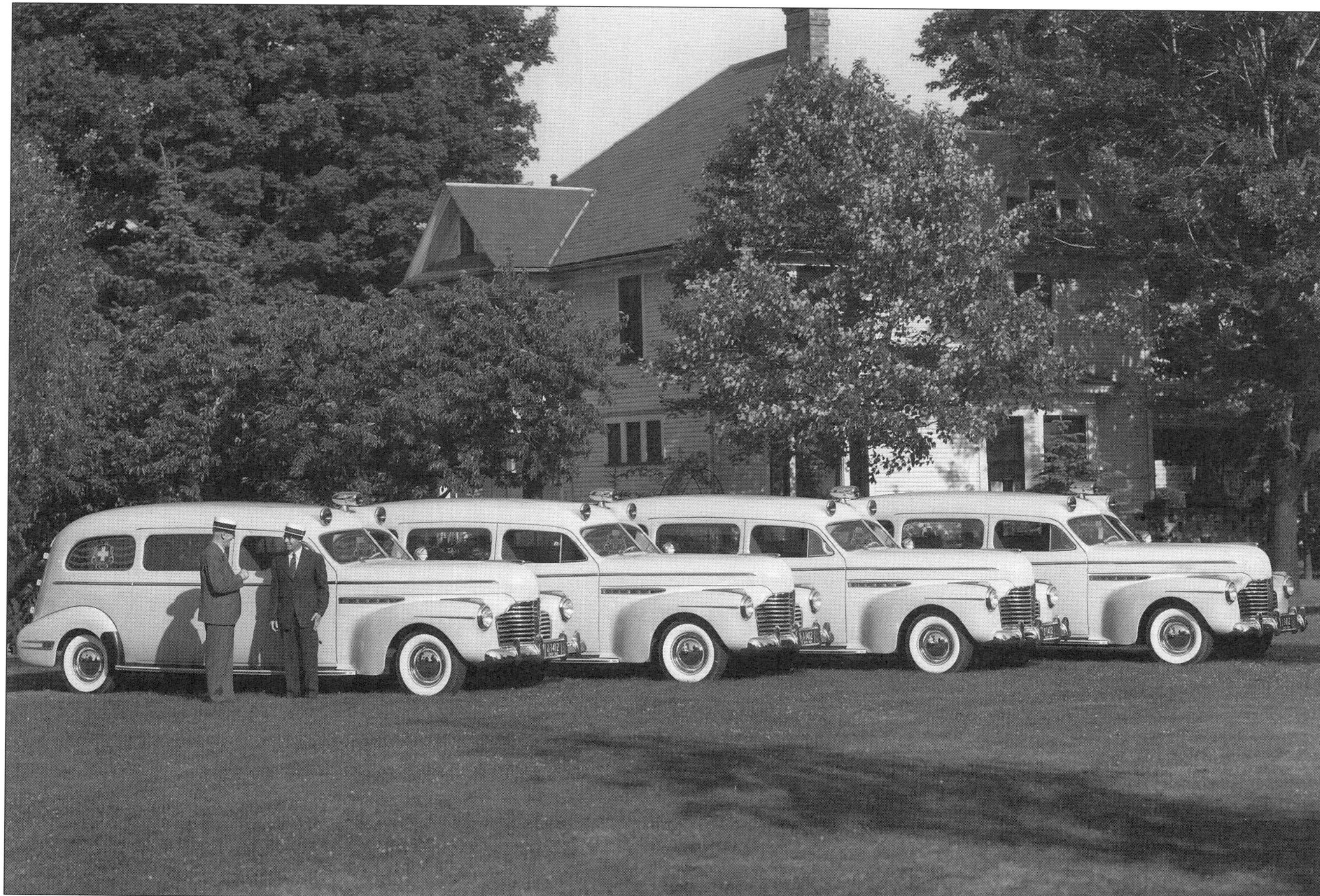

1941 FLXIBLE-BUICK AMBULANCE FLEET – As a customer courtesy, the Flxible Company photographer often took pictures of customers taking delivery of their new hearses and ambulances at the Loudonville, Ohio, plant. In this classic photo, a factory fresh fleet of four 1941 Flxible-Buick ambulances is turned over to its proud owners.

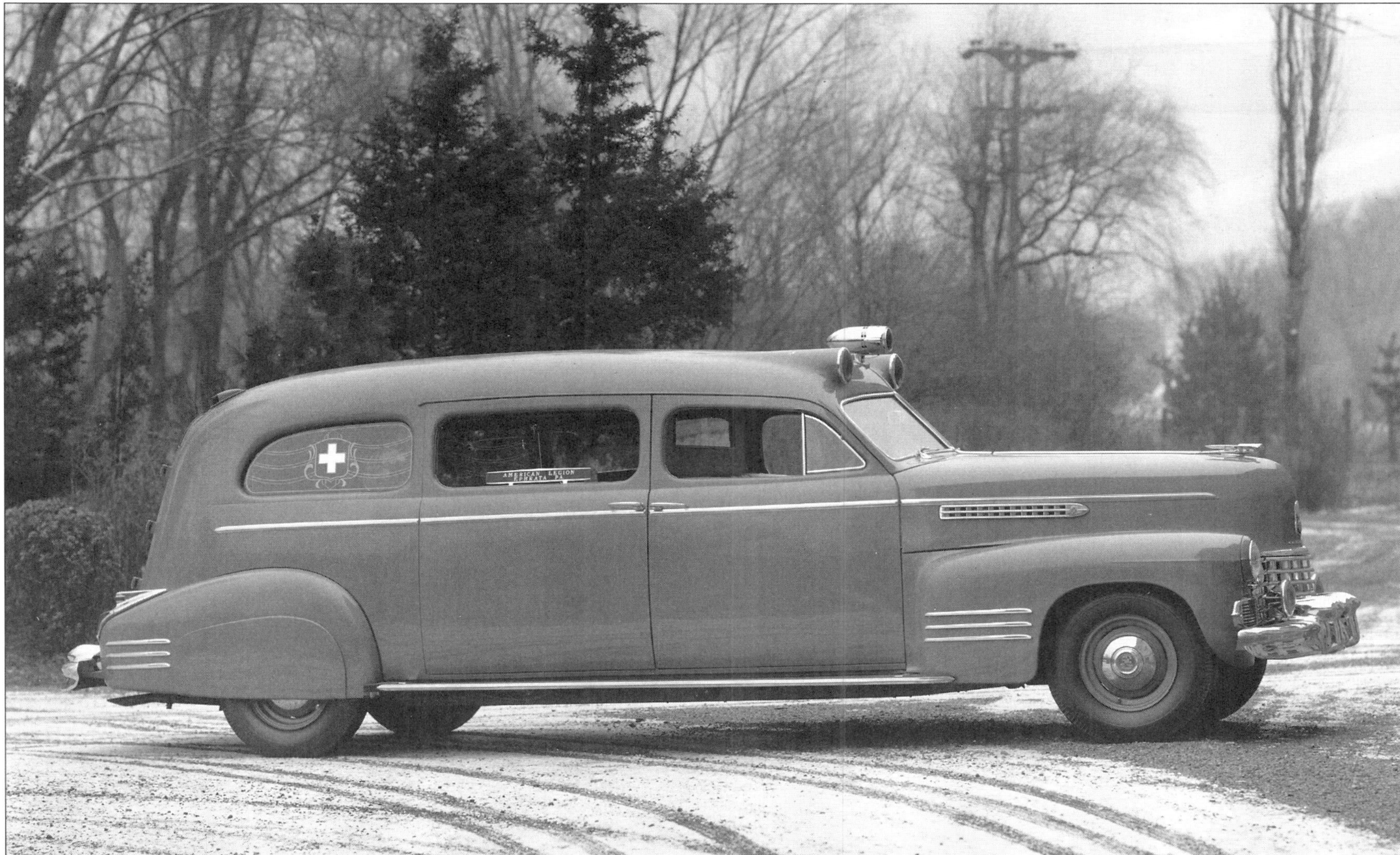

1942 FLXIBLE-CADILLAC AMBULANCE - The Flxible Company forged a strong alliance with the Buick Motor Division of General Motors dating back to the mid-1920s. Flxible mounted its hearse and ambulance bodies on Buick chassis almost exclusively from 1925 through 1938, when it also began to offer Cadillac and LaSalle professional cars. This arrangement was short-lived, however. After the war Flxible built on Buick chassis exclusively. This sturdy-looking 1942 Flxible-Cadillac Ambulance was built for the Ephrata, Pennsylvania Post of the American Legion.

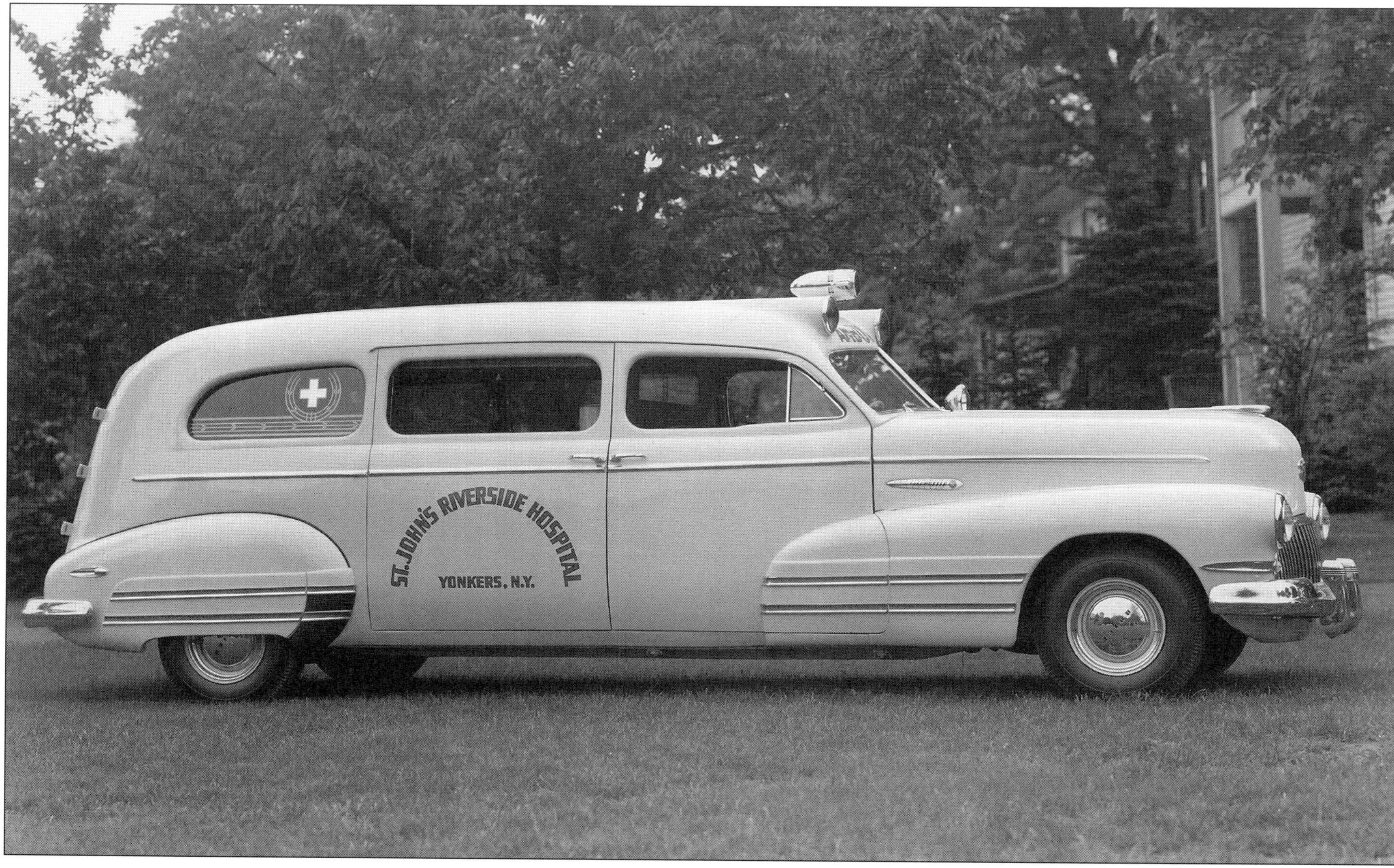

1942 FLXIBLE-BUICK AMBULANCE - Buick totally restyled its passenger cars for 1942. The new look featured "pontoon" fenders which flowed into the front doors. Thus Flxible was able to boast the only all-new professional car styling that year. This 1942 Flxible-Buick Ambulance was built for St. John's Riverside Hospital in Yonkers, New York. Business was good, but war clouds were gathering. After the attack on Pearl Harbor, American funeral car and ambulance manufacturers ceased production "for the duration" early in 1942.

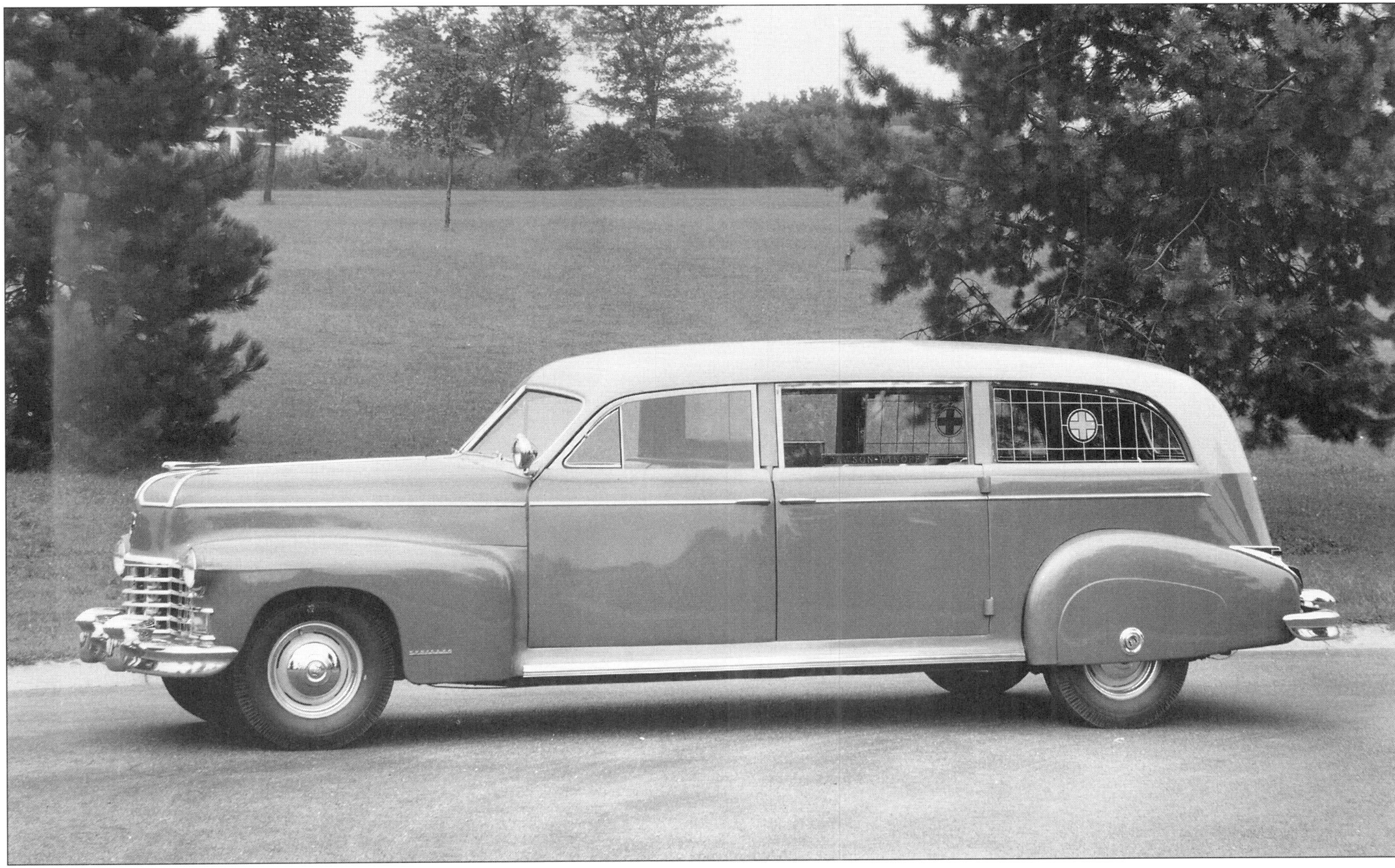

1946 S&S CADILLAC KENSINGTON AMBULANCE - American funeral car and ambulance production slowly resumed in 1945 following the end of the Second World War. Sayers & Scovill of Cincinnati was among the first to resume professional car production. Like all of the other manufacturers, S&S' 1946 models were basically warmed-over 1941-1942 designs. The Hess & Eisenhardt Co. had bought out Sayers and Scovill but continued to use the respected S&S name. Hearse, ambulance and limousine bodies complemented the angular architecture of the "senior" 1941-1949 Cadillacs.

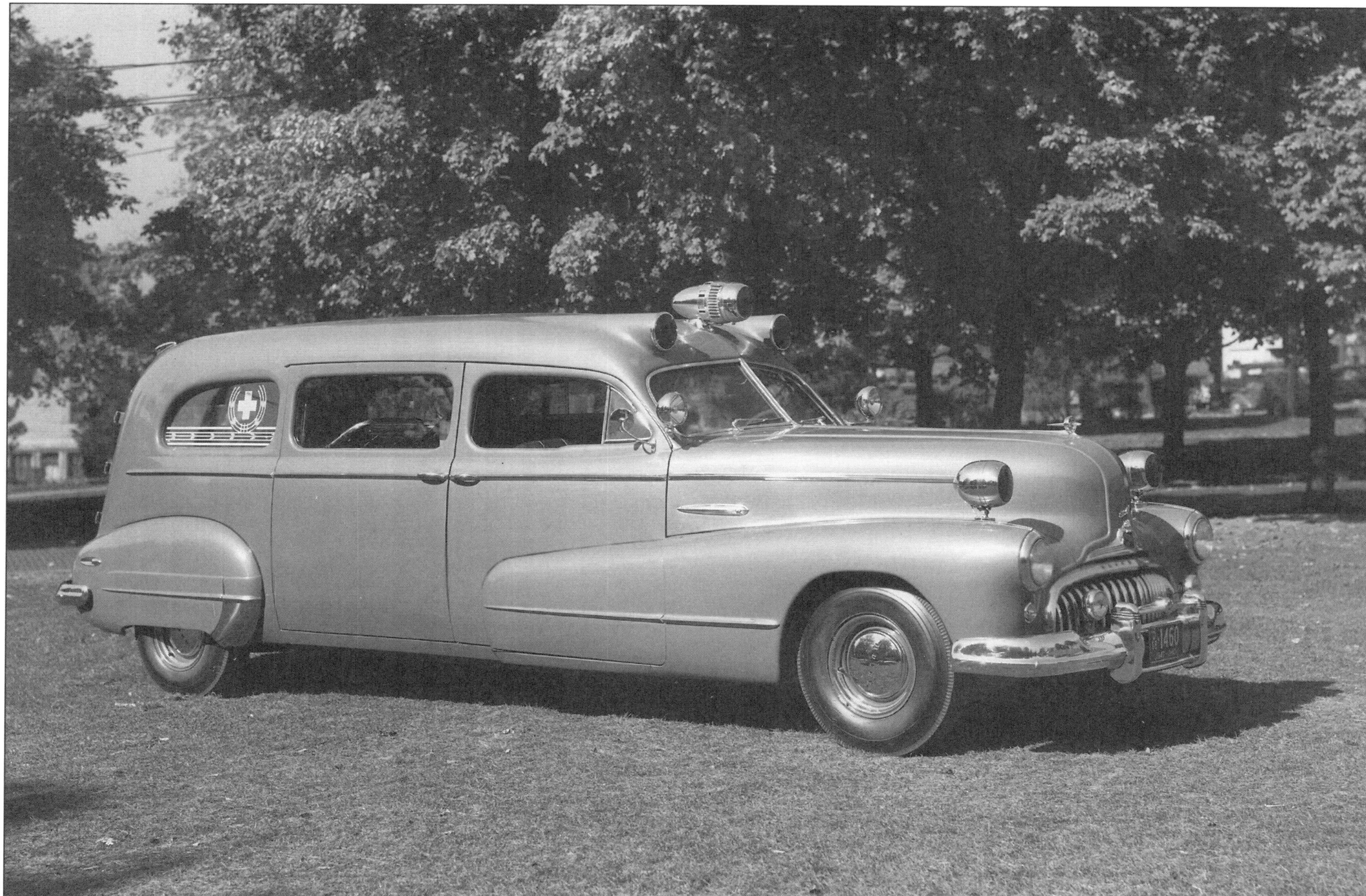

1947 FLXIBLE-BUICK AMBULANCE – The Flxible Co. built hundreds of Buick ambulances of this style between 1946 and 1948. This is a 1947 Flxible-Buick Premier Model B22-747 Ambulance. Extras include tunnel type roof lights, Federal Propello-Ray warning lights on both front fenders, a Federal C5 siren, fog lights and rear roof lights. Make no mistake about it, this was one *big* car!

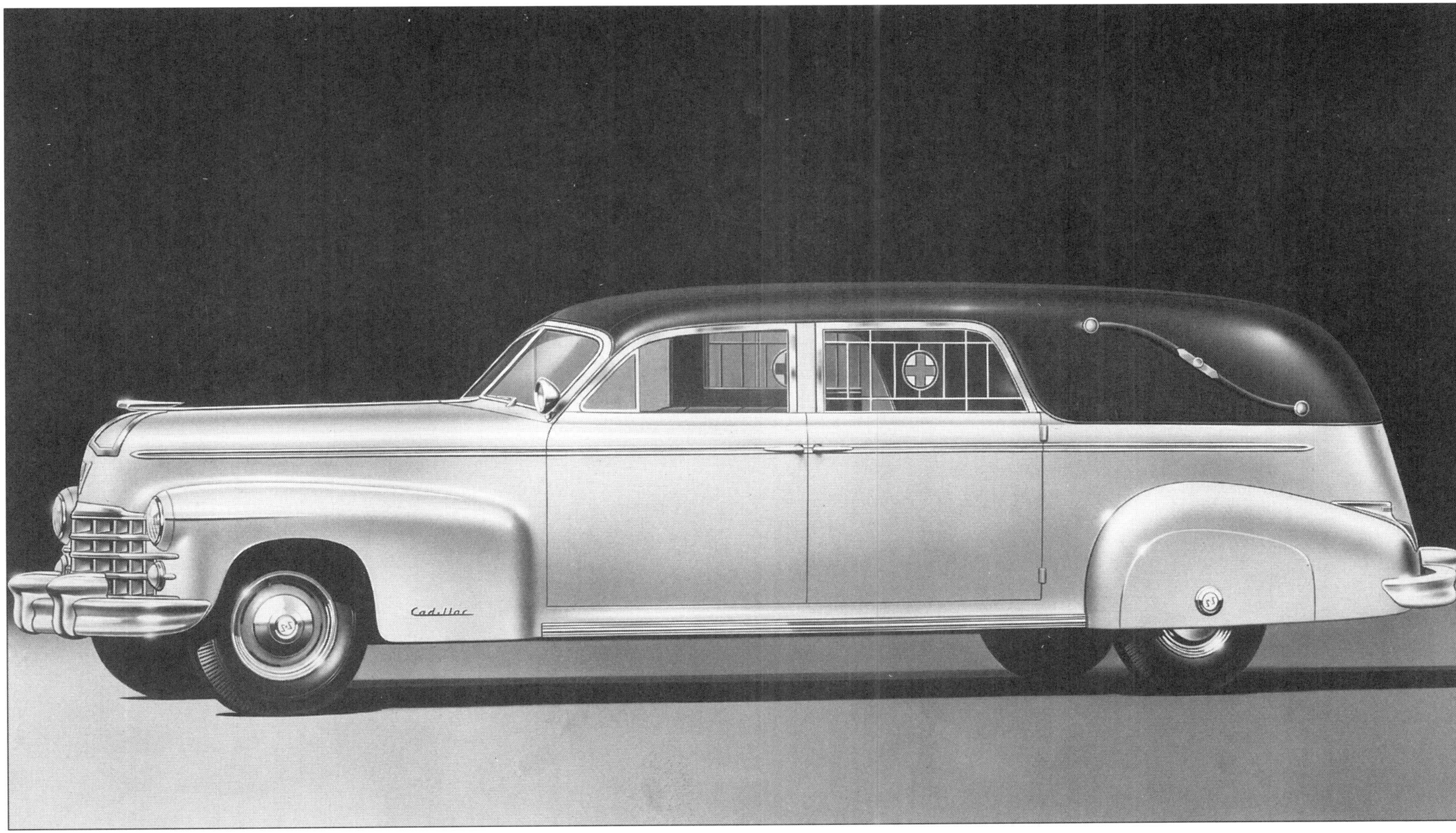

1947 S&S CADILLAC PARKWAY VICTORIA LANDAU AMBULANCE - Sayers & Scovill had introduced the Landau body style in 1938, with ornamental landau bows spanning large upper rear quarter panels. This is a catalog illustration of Hess & Eisenhardt's most stylish ambulance offering for 1948. In addition to formal landau styling, the 1947 S&S Cadillac Parkway Victoria features leaded glass ornamentation in its rear side door windows. This was the last year this holdover from the 1920s was offered by any ambulance manufacturer.

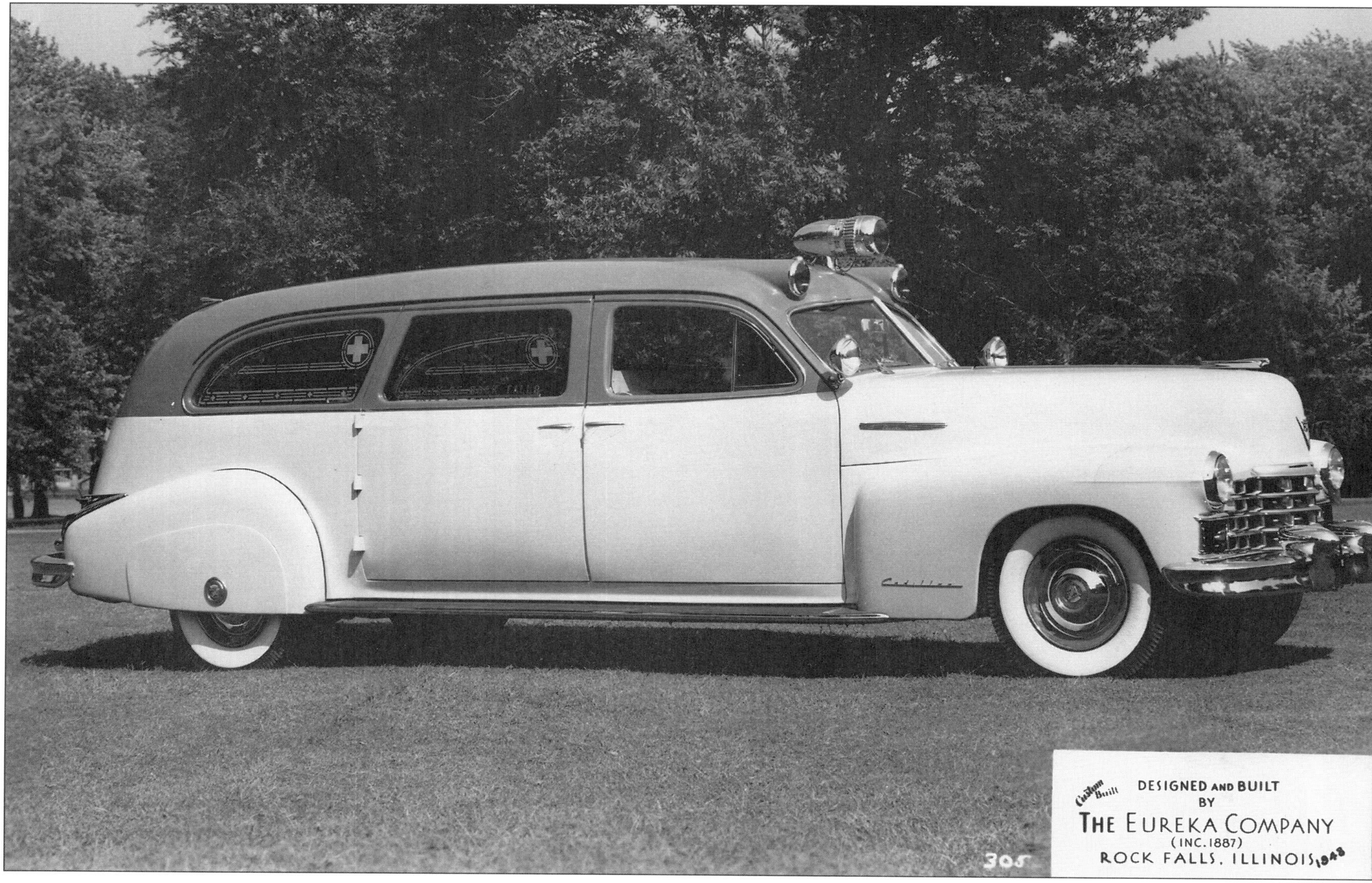
Custom Built
DESIGNED AND BUILT
BY
THE EUREKA COMPANY
(INC. 1887)
ROCK FALLS, ILLINOIS, 1948
305

1948 EUREKA-CADILLAC CHIEFTAIN AMBULANCE - Like rival Henney, The Eureka Company of Rock Falls, Illinois, switched from the dying buggy manufacturing business to building hearse and ambulance bodies in 1916. Eureka's modestly restyled postwar models featured an angled "C" body pillar, giving these cars a sleek, speedy look. The rear fender skirts also contributed to this car's clean appearance. On Eureka ambulances, red lenses replaced the standard parking light lenses at the outboard end of the massive Cadillac eggcrate grille.

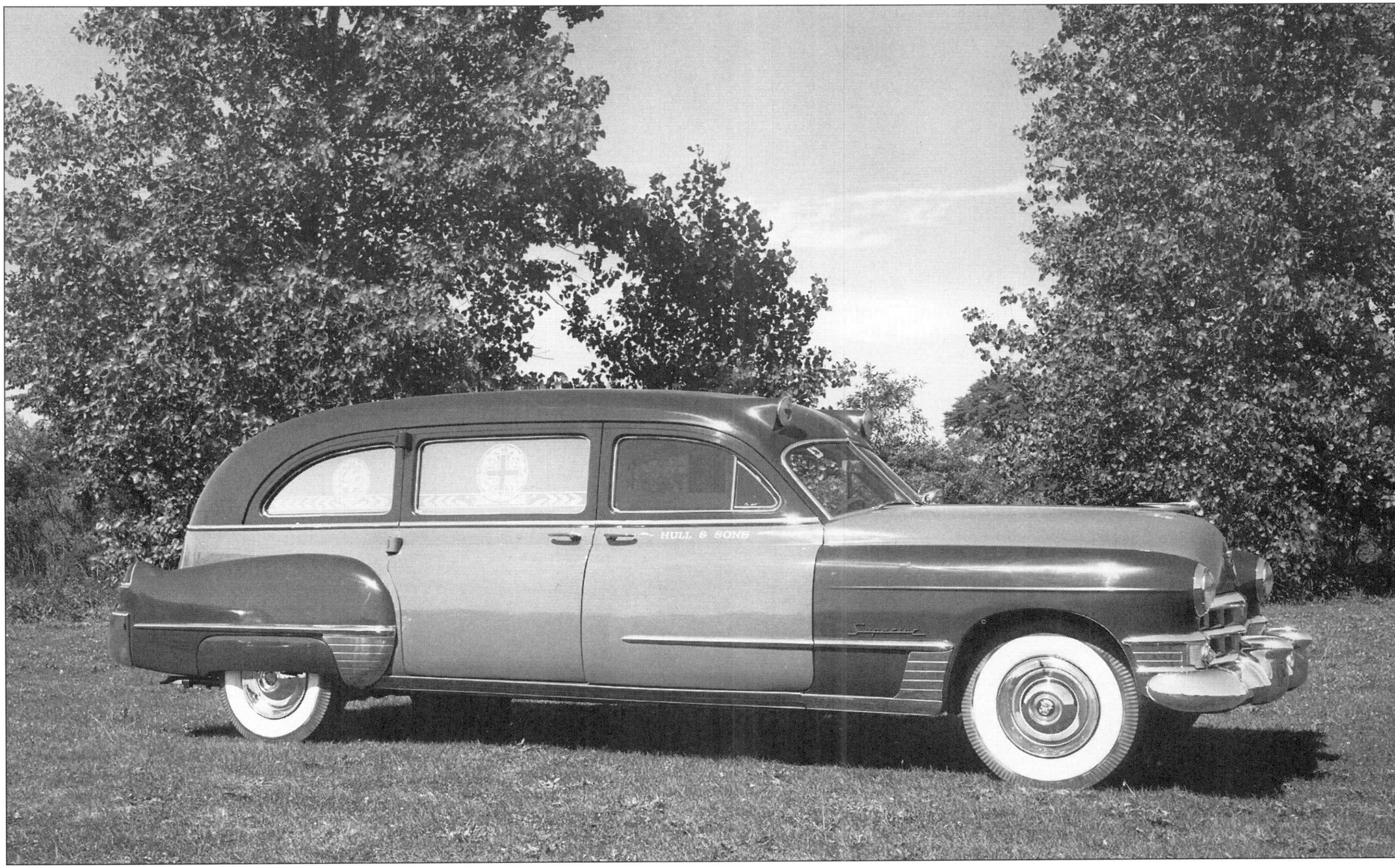

1949 SUPERIOR-CADILLAC AMBULANCE - The 1949 model year marked the introduction of Cadillac's first all-new postwar commercial chassis (although a small number of funeral cars and ambulances had been constructed on the all-new 1948 Cadillac, with its controversial "fishtail" fins). All of the major manufacturers — Superior, A. J. Miller, Meteor, Eureka and S&S — switched to the new Cadillac Series 86 commercial chassis for the 1949 model year. Only the companion Cadillac Fleetwood Seventy-Five Sedan and Limousine retained the now severely dated prewar Cadillac styling which had been introduced back in 1941.

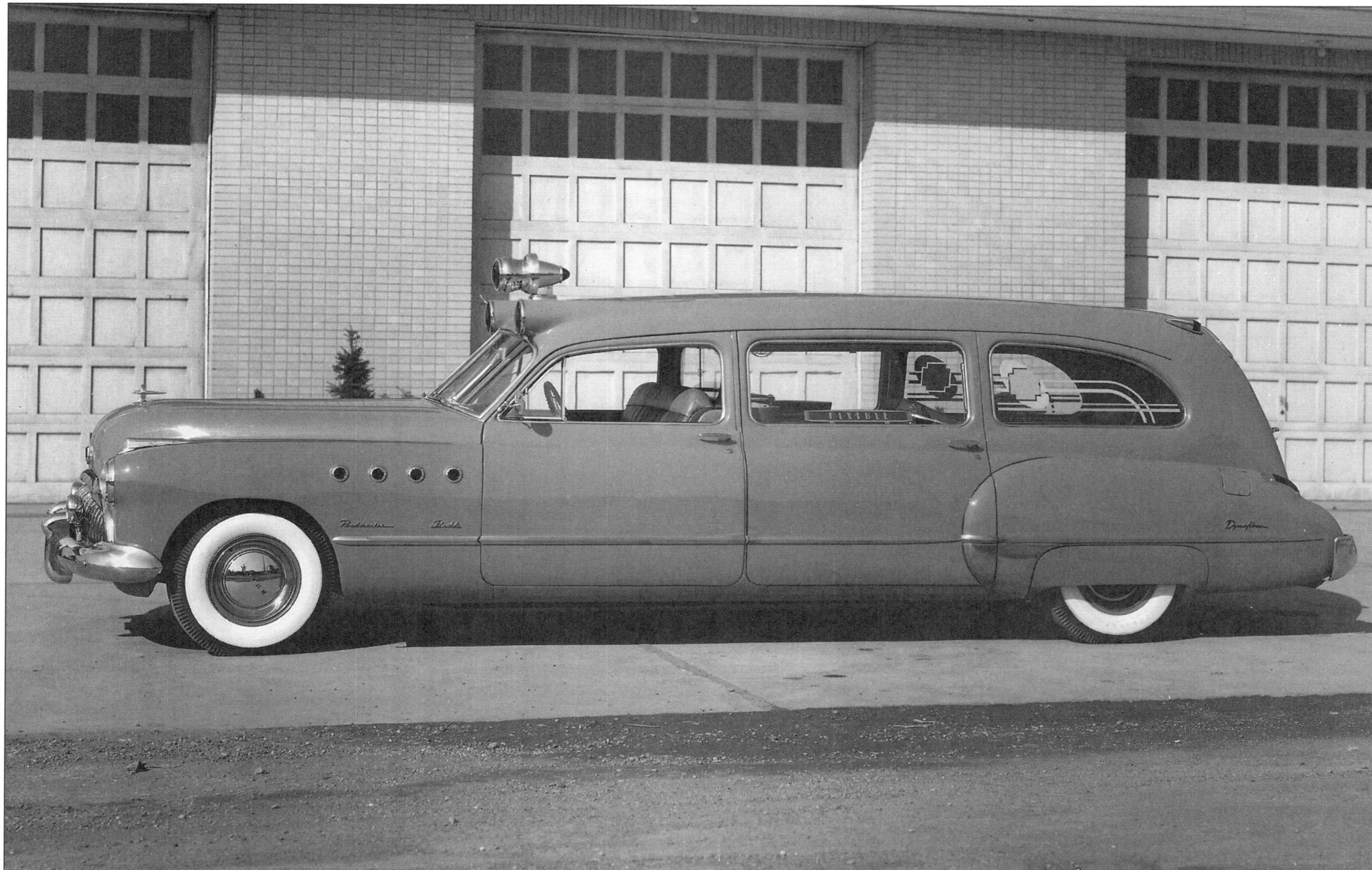

1949 FLXIBLE-BUICK PREMIER AMBULANCE – The Flxible Co. created a sensation with its all-new 1949 Buick professional cars. The new Flxibles were dramatically longer and lower — not only than the previous model Buicks that they replaced, but also its competitors' Cadillacs. This is the 1949 Flxible-Buick Model B22-749 Premier Ambulance. Options on this car include streamlined roof lights and the Sireno R5 siren on the roof.

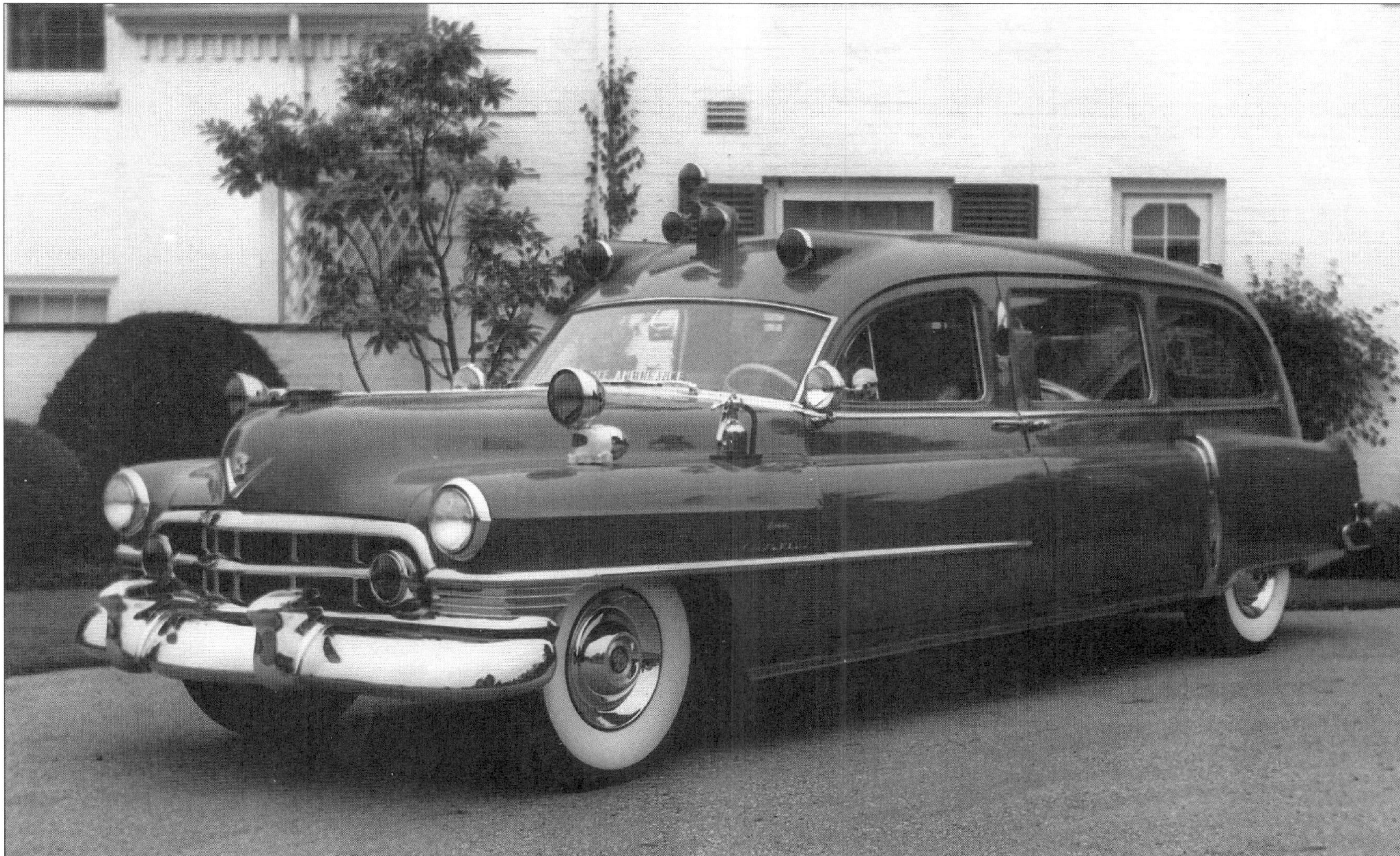

1950 METEOR-CADILLAC MODEL 501 AMBULANCE - For the second time in two years, the Cadillac commercial chassis was totally redesigned for 1950. The new Series 86 commercial chassis had Cadillac's massive new front-end ensemble with curved one-piece windshield. This very well equipped 1950 Meteor-Cadillac Ambulance is equipped with Mars wig-wag warning lights on each front fender, grille and tunnel roof light red flashers, Buckeye Roto-Rays and a C02 fire extinguisher mounted in the left front fender. The large coach lamps mounted on the front doors were a trademark of the Meteor Motor Car Company of Piqua, Ohio.

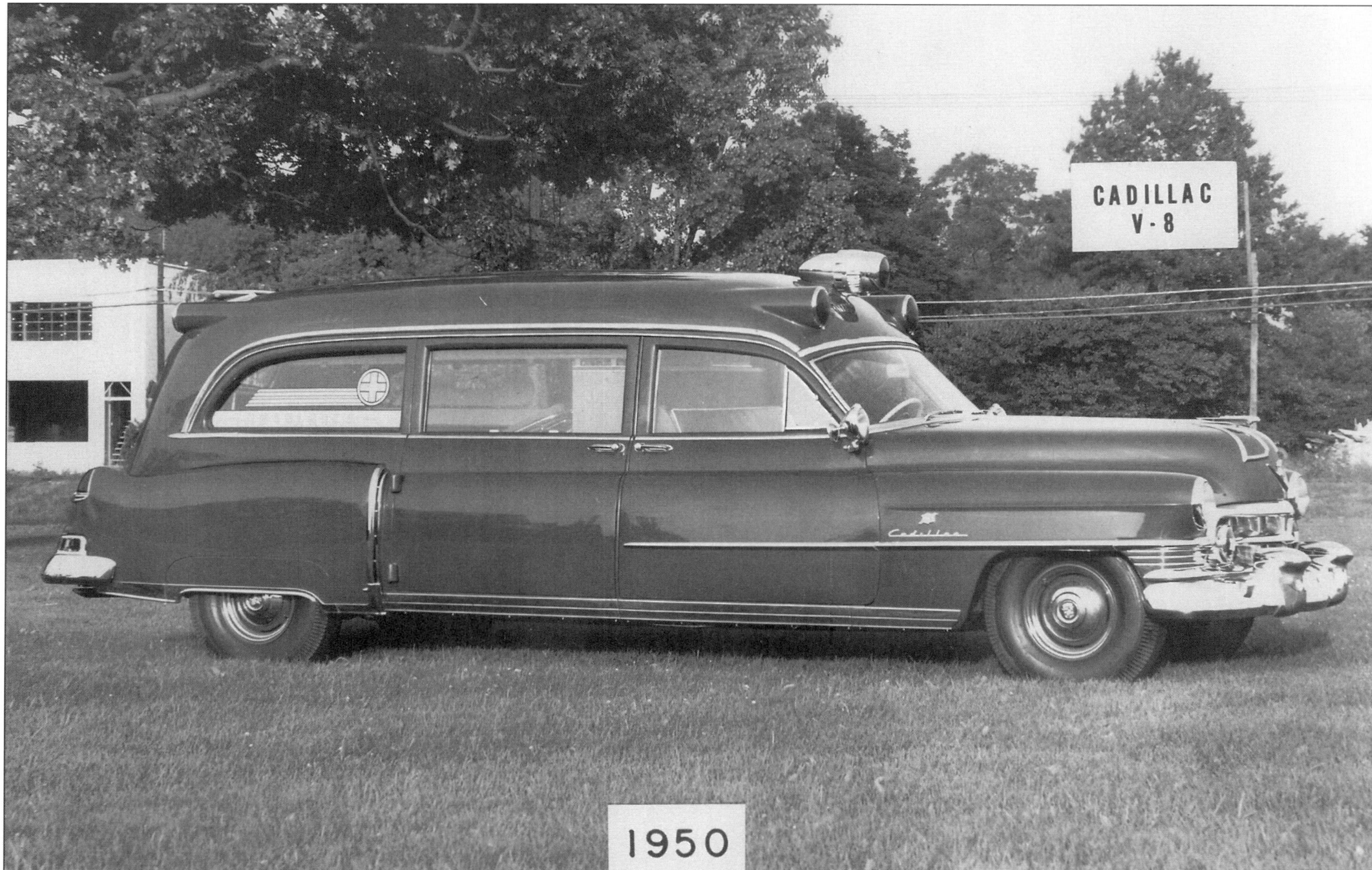

1950 S&S CADILLAC HIGHTOP AMBULANCE - High headroom ambulances capable of comfortably accommodating four litter patients had been custom-built by several ambulance manufacturers since the late 1930s. Sayers & Scovill had delivered one to the Cincinnati General Hospital in 1939. Raised-roof, high-headroom ambulances became standard industry offerings in the 1950s. Note the "tunneled" roof warning lights front and rear, and the distinctive S&S chrome trim on the leading edge of this car's hood.

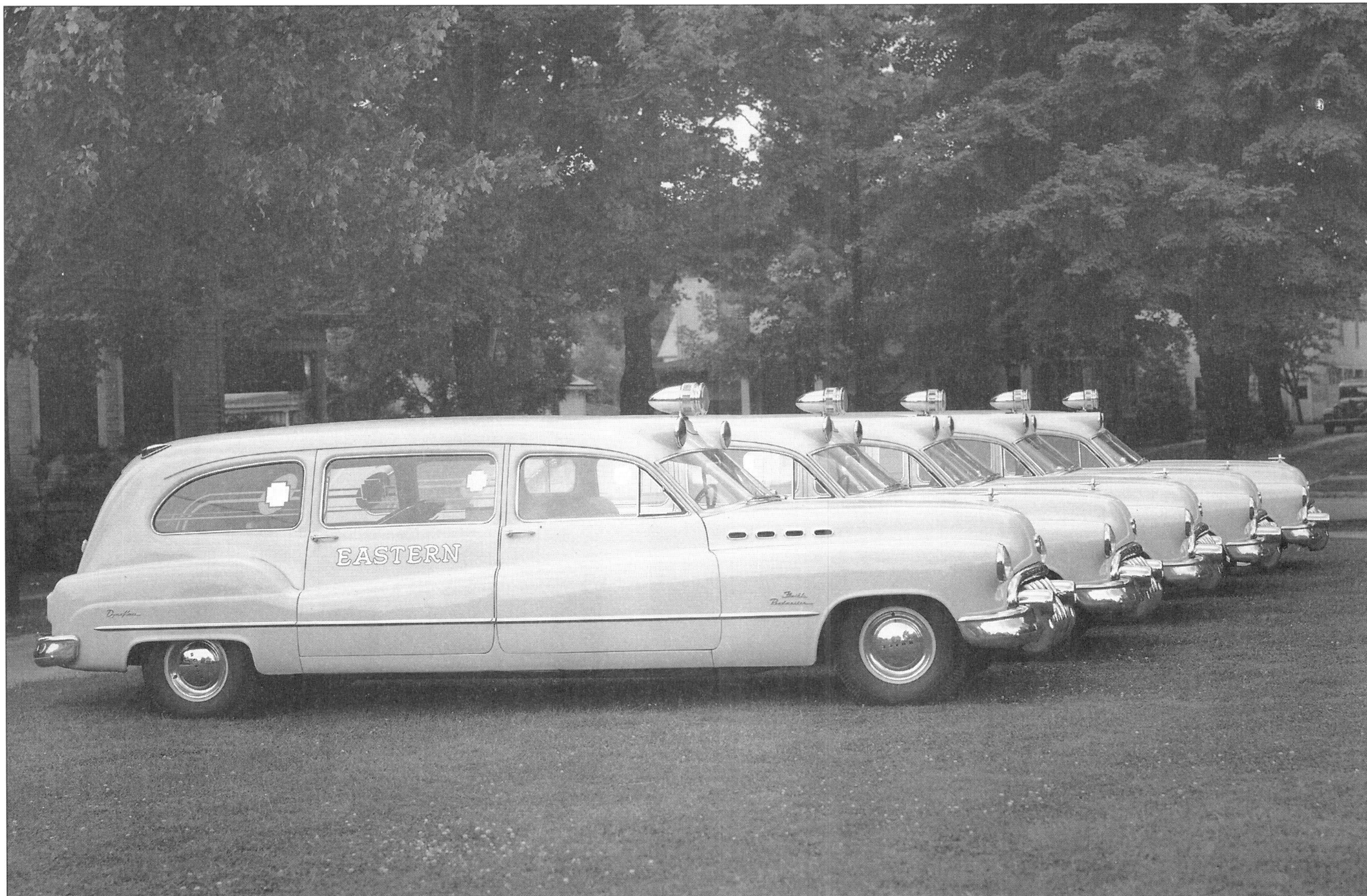

1950 FLXIBLE-BUICK AMBULANCE FLEET - The Flxible Co. delivered this fleet of five Flxible-Buick Premier ambulances to Eastern Ambulance, a large East Coast ambulance operator. The top-line Flxible Premier was built on the Buick Roadmaster chassis. The less expensive Flxible Sterling Ambulance was built on the Buick Special chassis that had three (instead of four) of Buick's distinctive hood "ventiports."

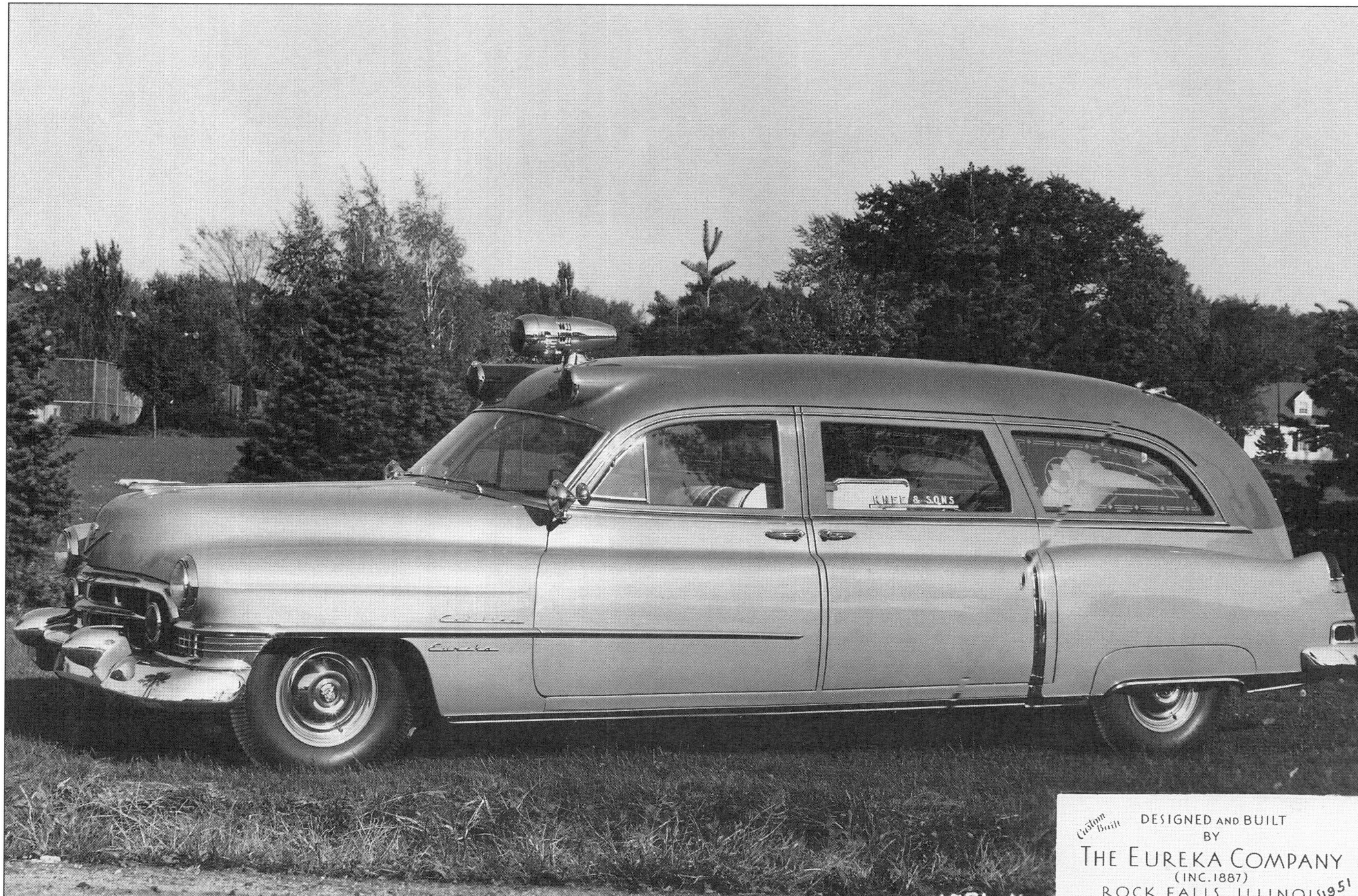

1951 EUREKA-CADILLAC AMBULANCE - Built on the 1951 Cadillac Series 86 commercial chassis, this standard model Eureka-Cadillac Limousine Ambulance features a two-tone paint job and black sidewall tires. Note the roof-mounted Federal C6 Duo-Tone siren. Alternating red flashing lights are built into the outboard ends of the grille and incorporated into the “tunnel” roof lights.

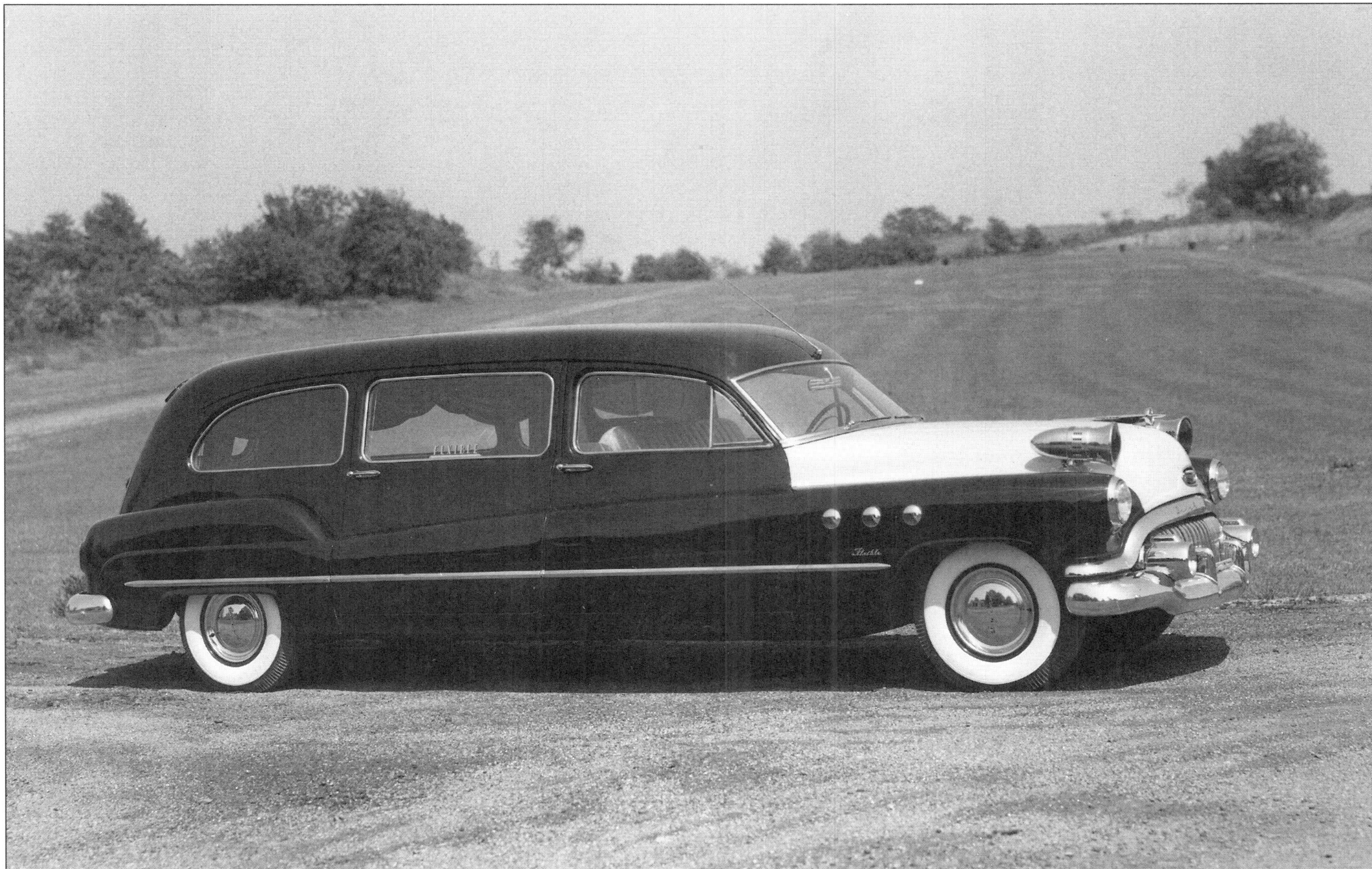

1951 FLXIBLE-BUICK COMBINATION - Built on the Buick Super chassis, this 1951 Flxible-Buick Sterling Combination Funeral Car/Ambulance sports one of the most unique options offered by Flxible: an extra hood. When this car was used as an ambulance, the standard black hearse hood was replaced with a white-painted hood equipped with two Sterling 30 sirens. An optional hood with faired-in red flashing lights was also available.

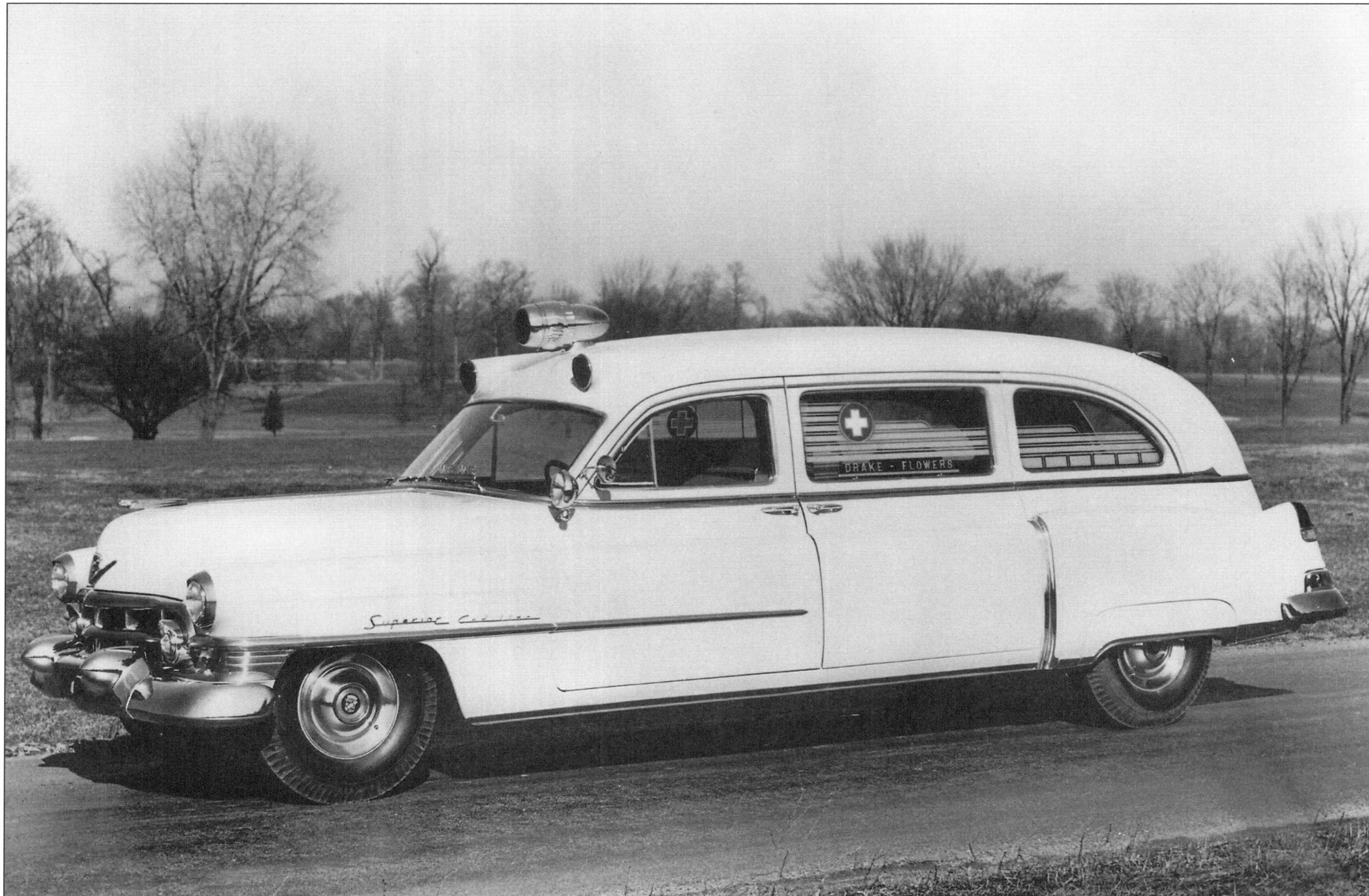

1952 SUPERIOR-CADILLAC LIMOUSINE AMBULANCE - Built for the Drake-Flowers Funeral Home, this white-painted straight ambulance had a factory drive away price of $7,167.00. Warning equipment included a Federal C6 siren and tunnel roof lights. Standard ambulance equipment included a remote-control spotlight and etched glass in the rear side windows for privacy, and to identify the car as an emergency vehicle.

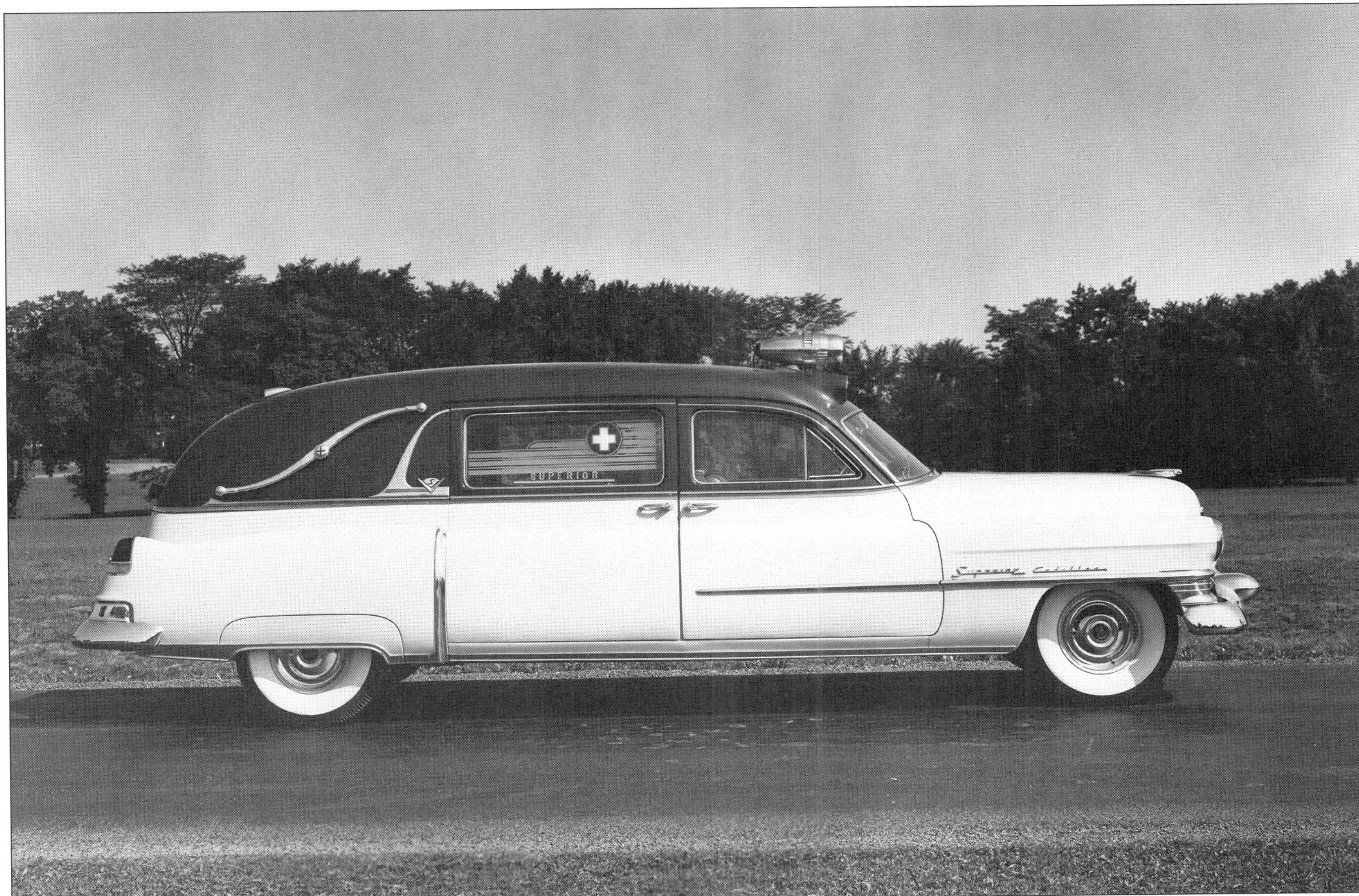

1952 SUPERIOR-CADILLAC LANDAULET AMBULANCE - The most prestigious ambulance Superior offered was the stately Superior-Cadillac Landaulet. Formal styling features included closed upper rear quarter panels ornamented with chrome landau bows. Other stylish touches include distinctive two-tone paint and white sidewall tires. The Superior-Cadillac Landaulet Ambulance sold for $7,400.00.

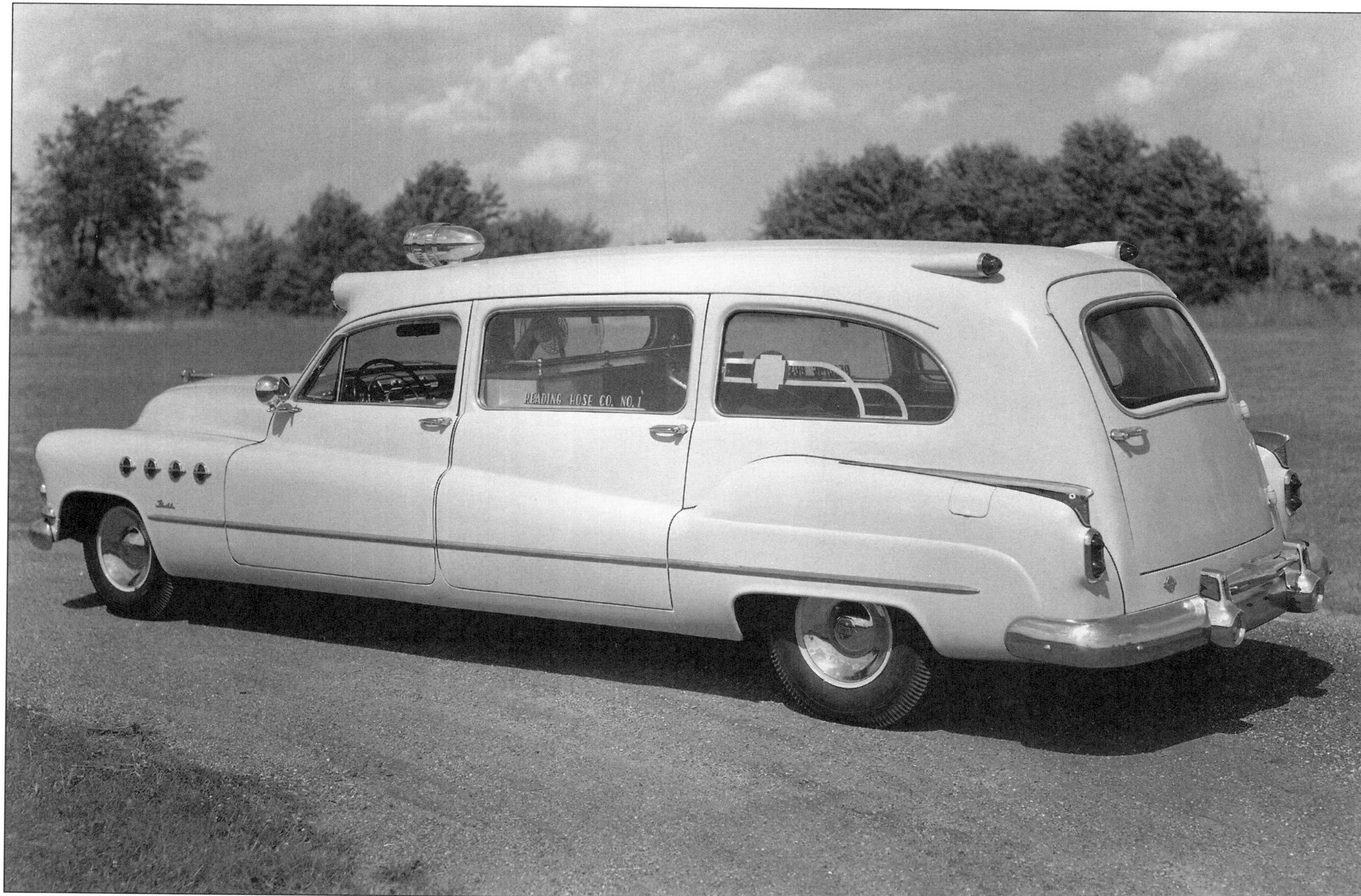

1952 FLXIBLE-BUICK PREMIER AMBULANCE - This sleekly styled limousine ambulance on Buick Roadmaster chassis was built for the Reading Hose Co. No. 1 of Reading, Pennsylvania. Note the red-lensed "bullet" lights on the rear roof. The Flxible Co. ceased funeral car and ambulance production at the end of the 1952 model year, but returned to the professional car field seven years later.

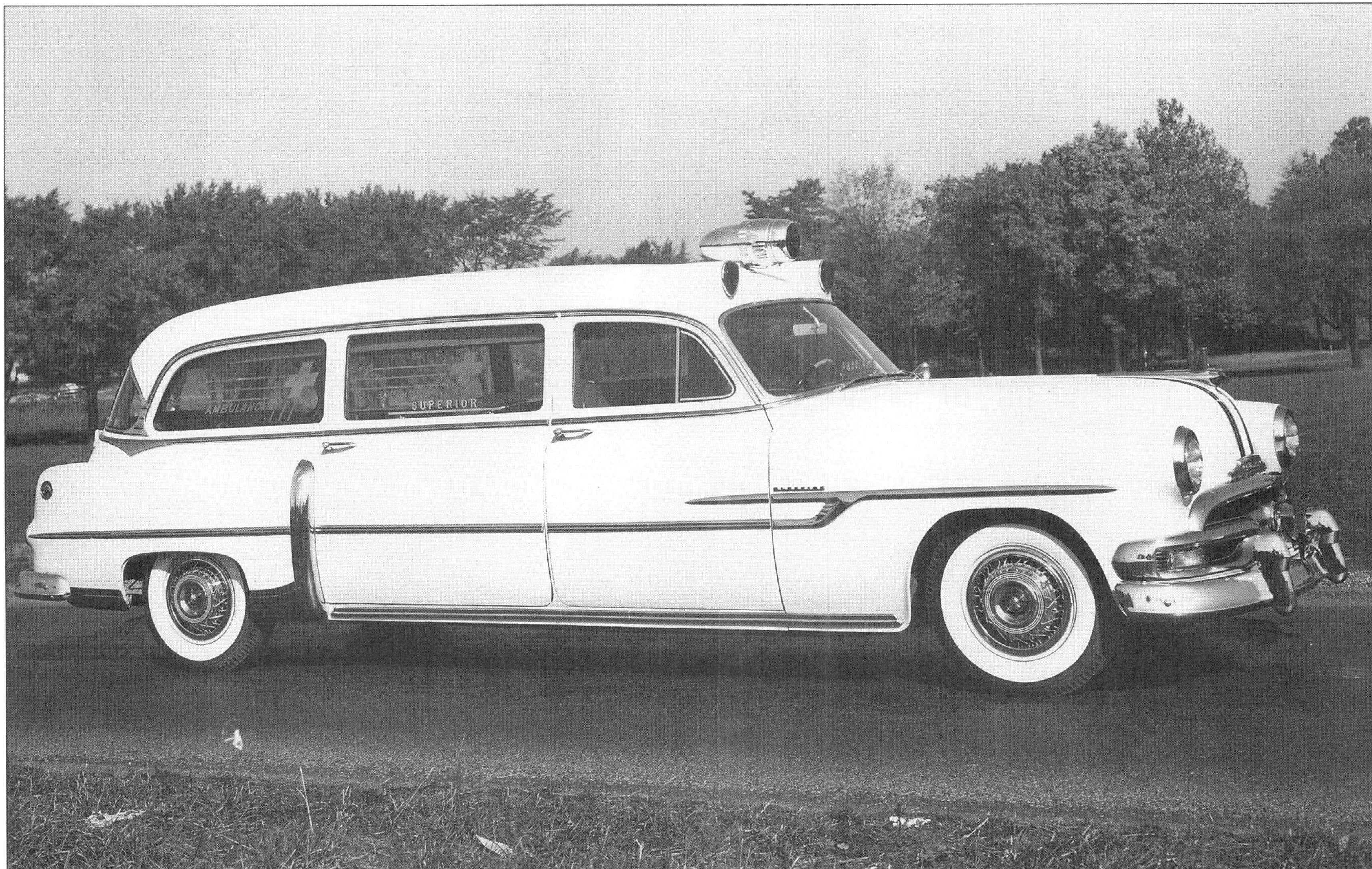

1953 SUPERIOR-PONTIAC AMBULANCE - After an absence of four years, Superior Coach re-entered the moderately priced ambulance field in 1953. The all-new Superior-Pontiac funeral cars and ambulances were built on stretched Pontiac Chieftain chassis in Superior's new Southern Division plant in Kosiusko, Mississippi, where they would continue to be sourced for the next 22 years. This 1953 Superior-Pontiac Ambulance sports wire wheel covers and the trendy new rear quarter windows.

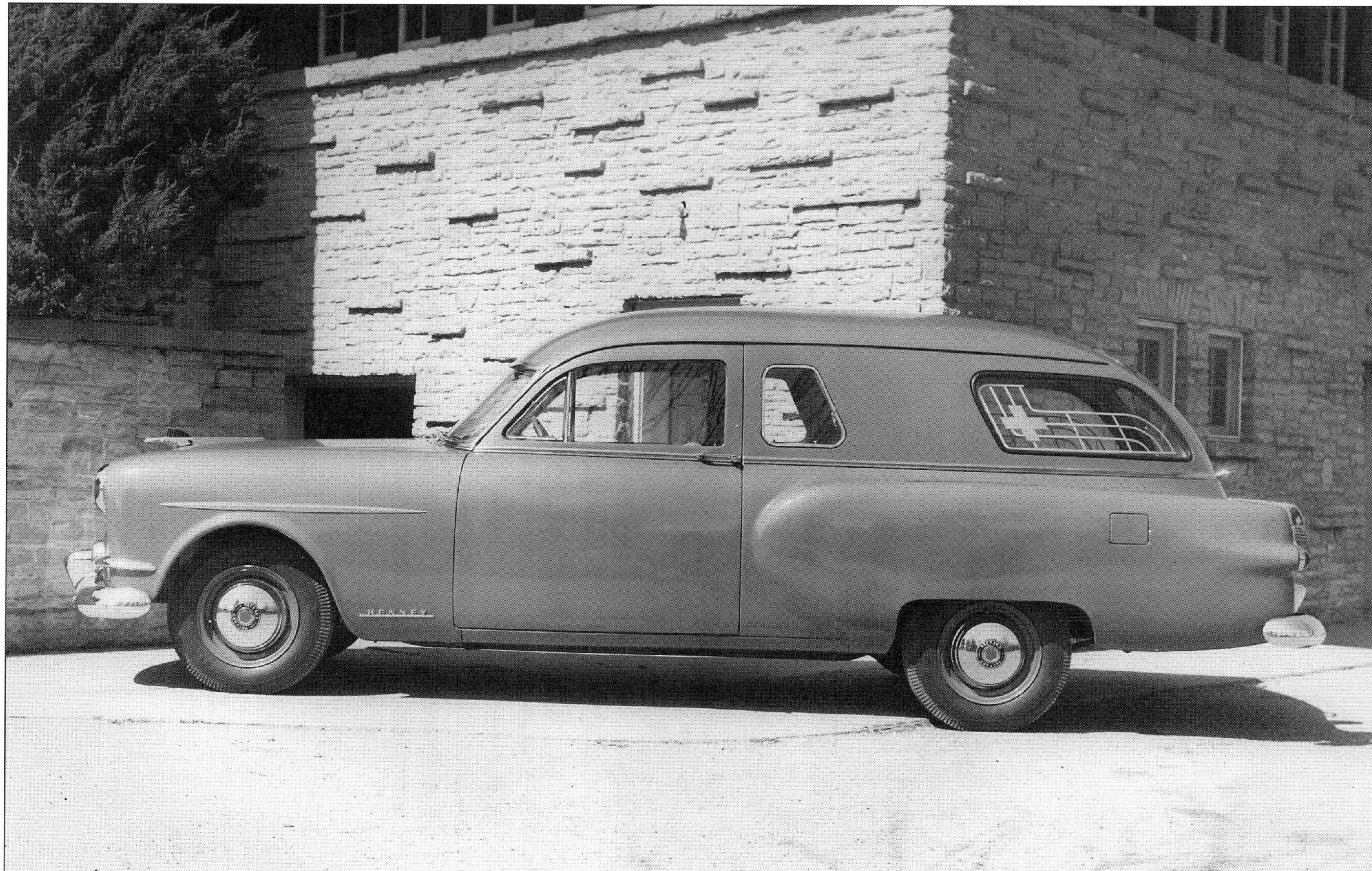

1953 HENNEY-PACKARD "JUNIOR" AMBULANCE - In 1951, the Henney Motor Company announced a new series of budget-priced "compact" professional cars. Built in ambulance, funeral car and combination variants, the Henney Junior was built on a standard-wheelbase Packard Clipper chassis with a raised roof. Seriously underpriced, the Henney Junior was a money-losing proposition for its maker. The versatile Junior died with Henney at the end of the 1954 model year.

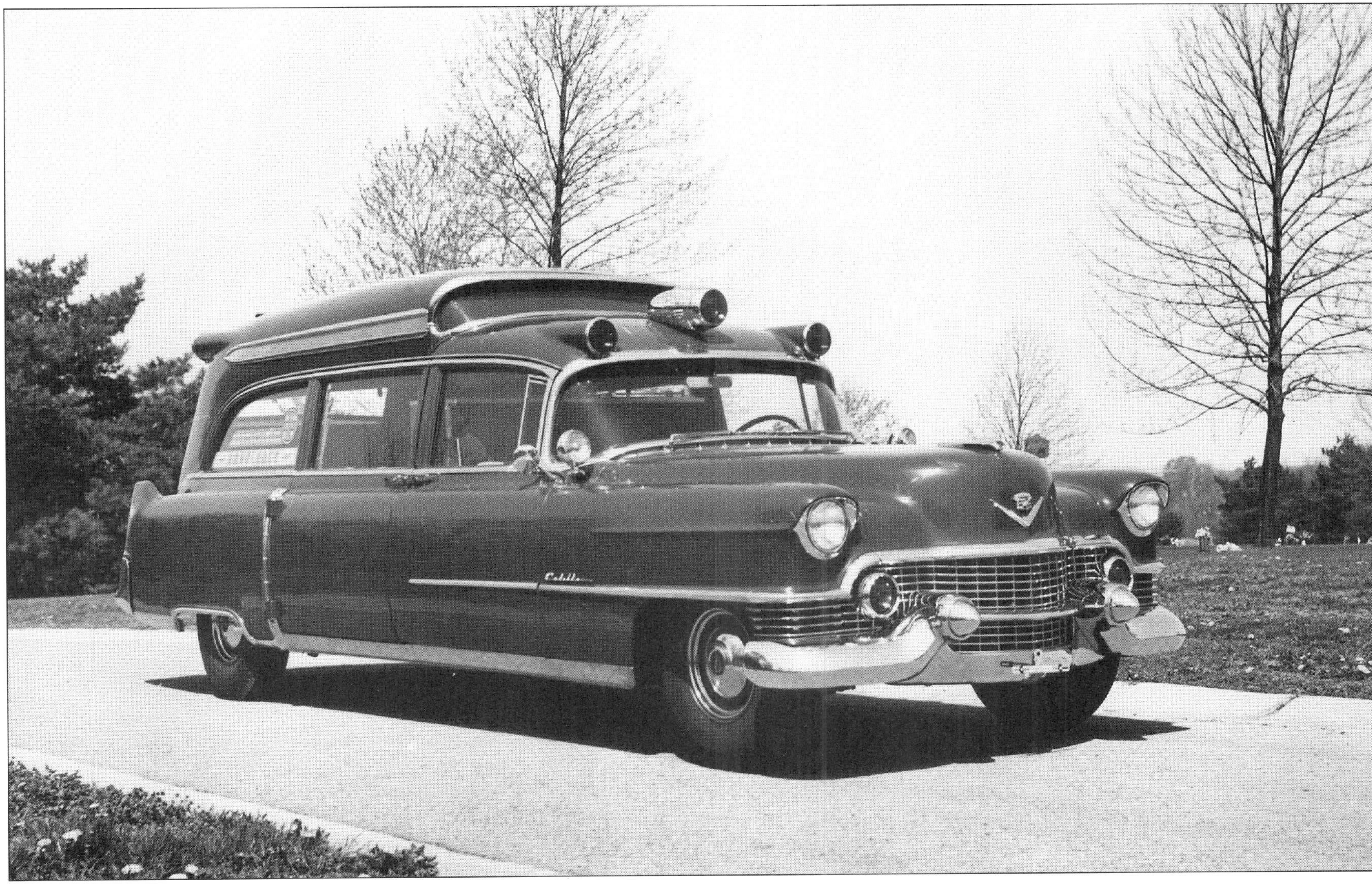

1954 S&S CADILLAC HIGHTOP AMBULANCE - The rescue type, raised-roof ambulance was steadily gaining in favor with professional ambulance operators. The Hess & Eisenhardt Co., builders of S&S professional cars, complemented its standard headroom Kensington Limousine Ambulance with the raised-roof S&S Professional Kensington in 1950. This is the 1954 S&S Cadillac Professional Kensington. The red plastic panel on the leading edge of the raised rear roof was illuminated.

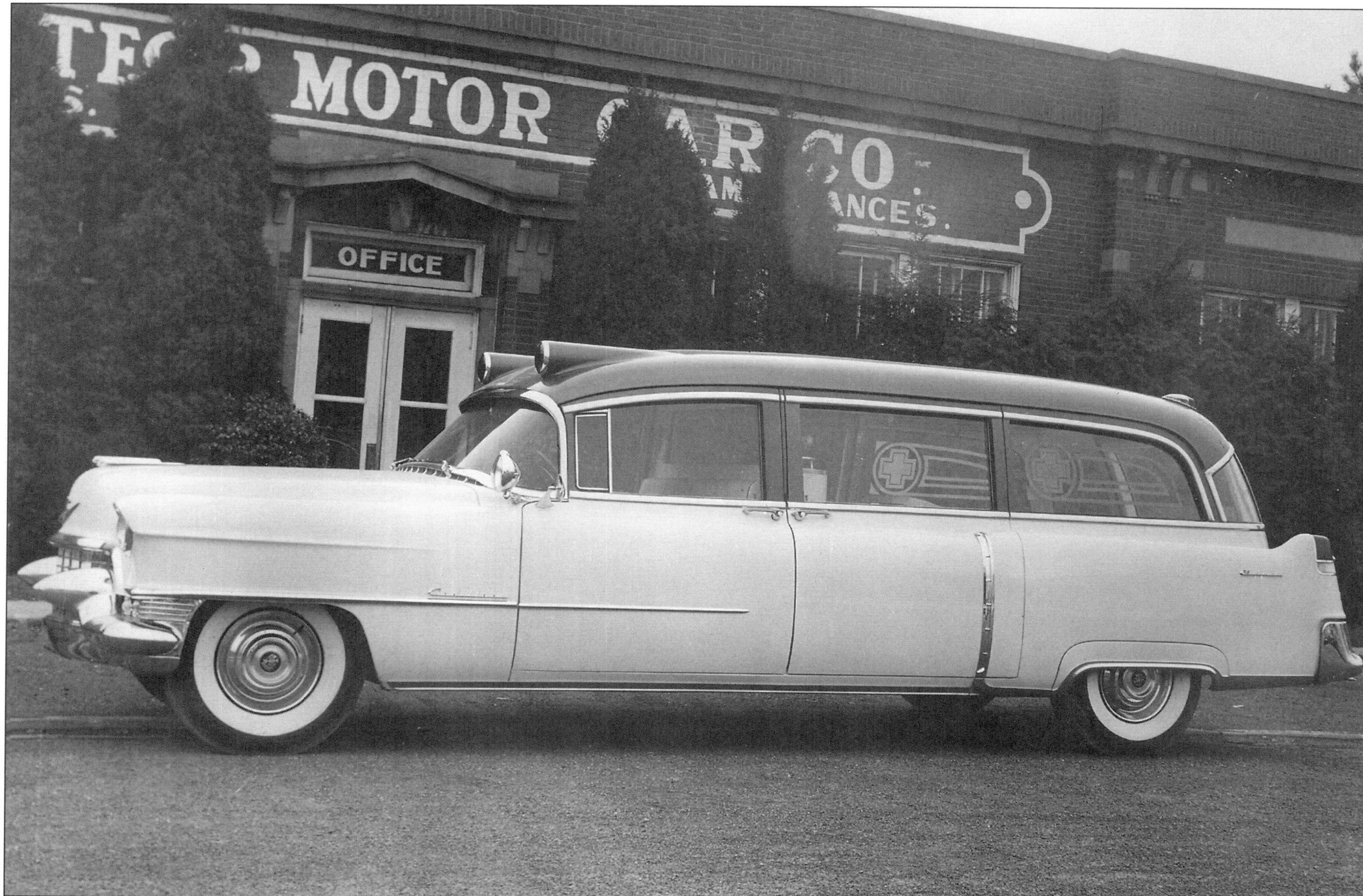

1955 METEOR-CADILLAC AMBULANCE - Posed in front of the Meteor Motor Car Company office in Piqua, Ohio, is a factory-fresh 1955 Meteor-Cadillac Limousine Ambulance. Note the handsome two-tone paint job, tunnel-type roof lights and etched glass in the rear quarter windows. This sleek, lifesaving beauty was equipped with an underhood siren.

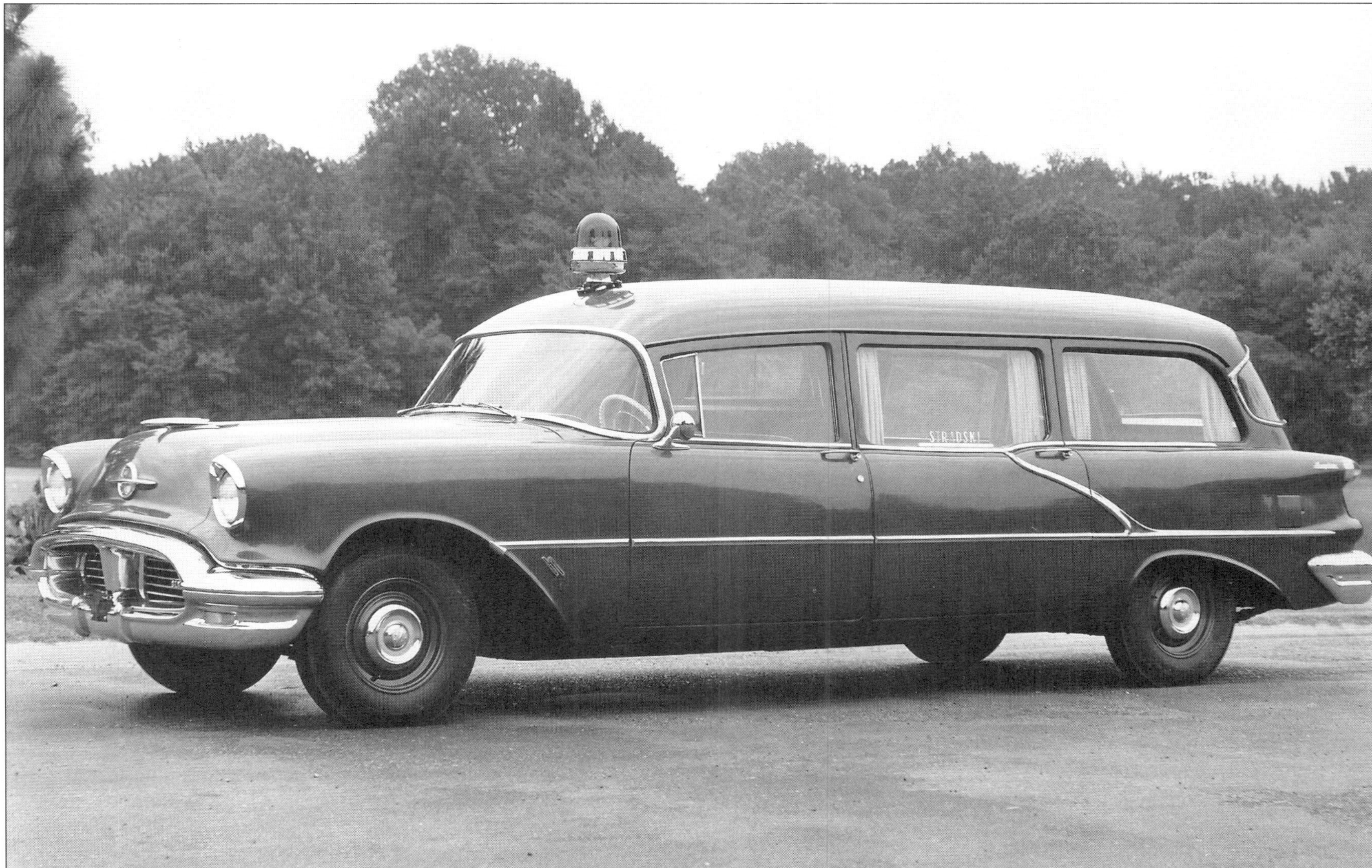

1955 MEMPHIAN-OLDSMOBILE AMBULANCE - The Memphis Coach Company was one of three Memphis, Tennessee, firms (Memphian, Economy and Weller) which specialized in funeral car and ambulance conversions of standard passenger cars. Memphian built ambulances on virtually any chassis desired by the customer. This good-looking Memphian Combination Funeral Coach & Ambulance was built on a lengthened 1955 Oldsmobile 88 chassis. Note the post-mounted Federal Beacon Ray warning light on the roof.

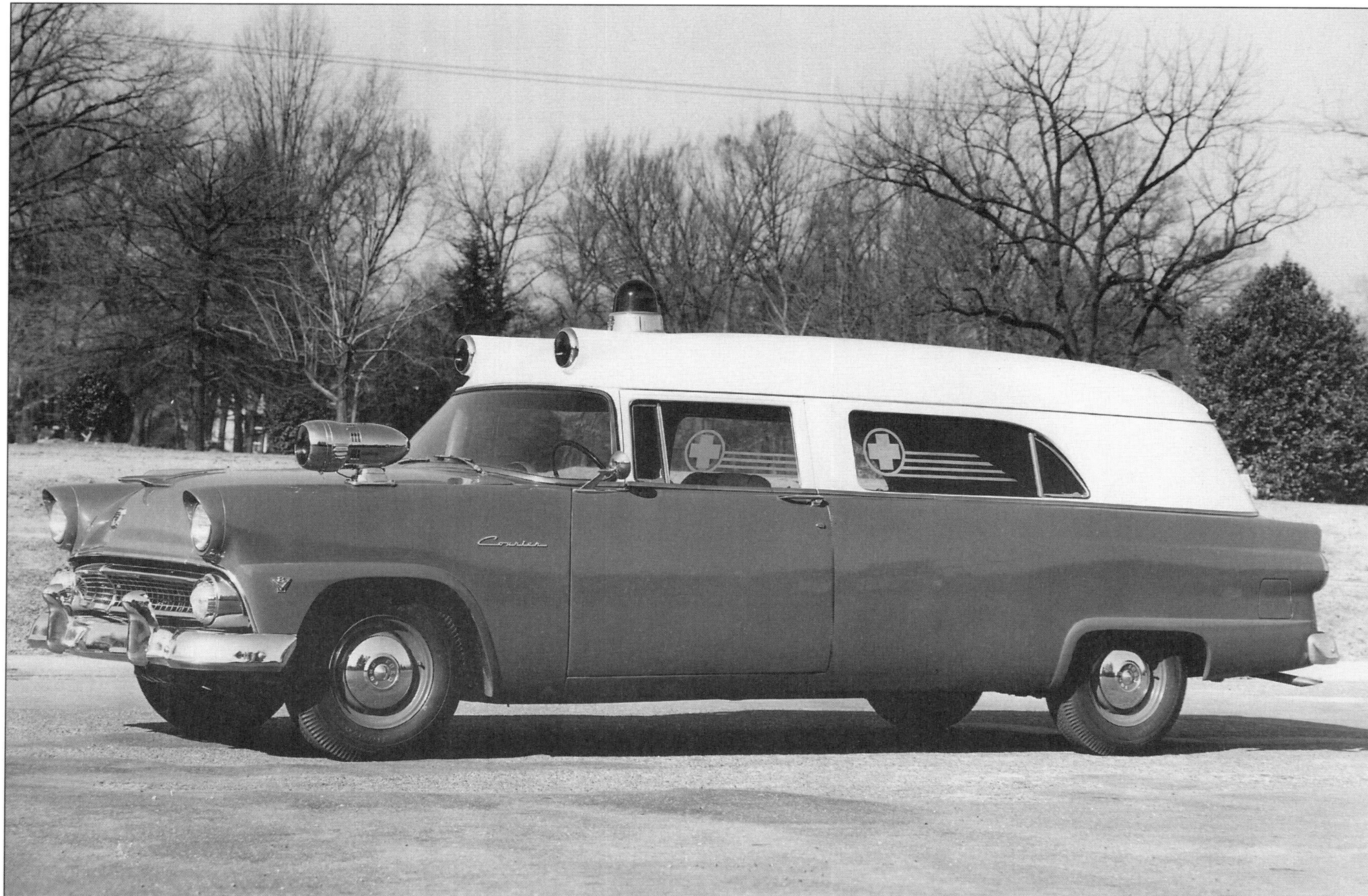

1955 MEMPHIAN-FORD JUNIOR AMBULANCE - The Memphis Coach Company built this straight ambulance conversion of a 1955 Ford Courier Sedan Delivery. Overall length was stretched 22 inches. For a budget-priced small town ambulance, this unit sports some decidedly "big city" warning devices: a lusty Federal C6 siren mounted on the left front fender and a roof-mounted Federal Beacon Ray.

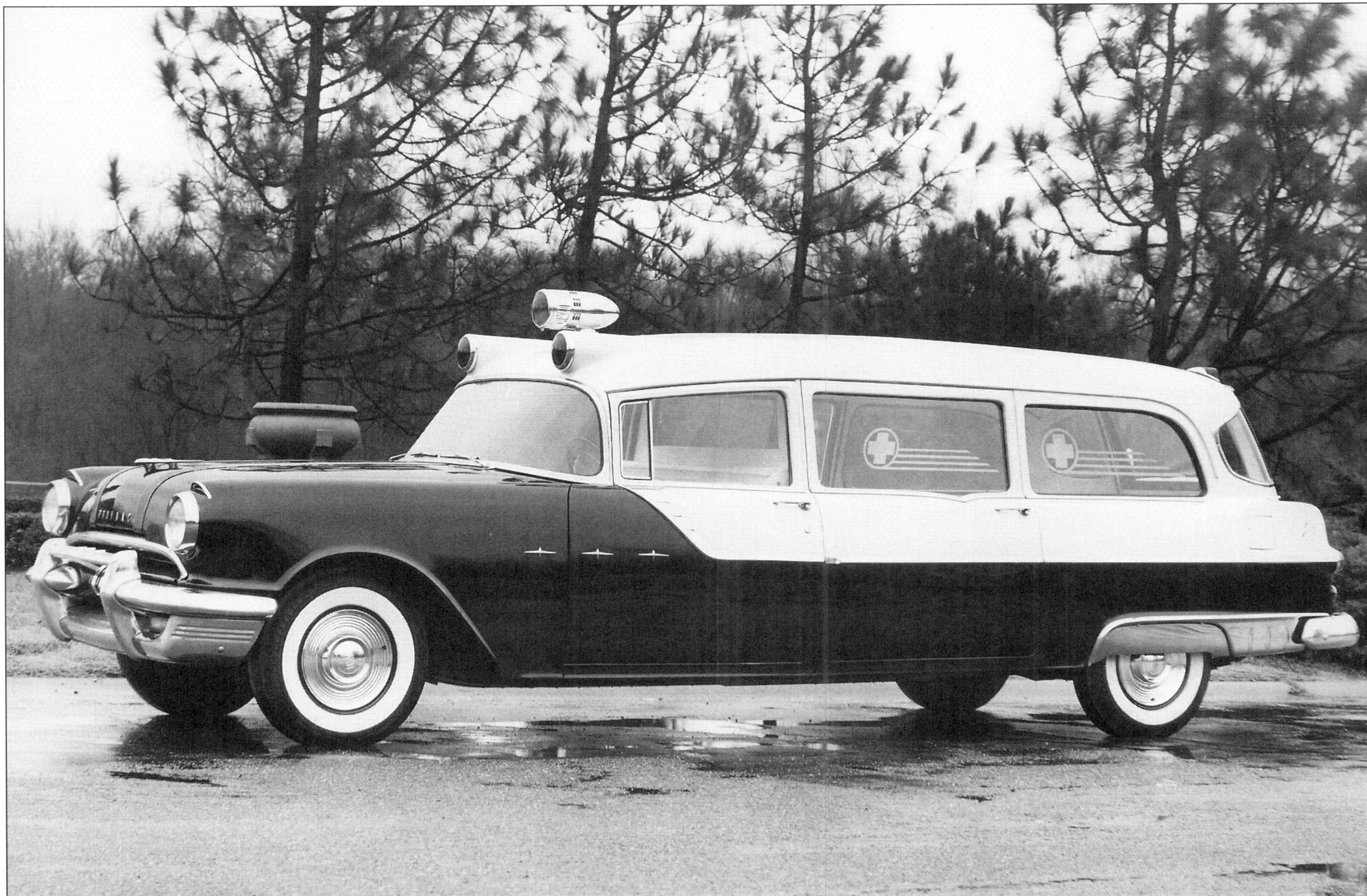

1955 ECONOMY-PONTIAC AMBULANCE - Predecessor to the Memphis Coach Co., the Economy Coach Company of Memphis, Tennesee, built this 1955 Economy-Pontiac Style 862 Straight Ambulance. Attractive styling features include two-tone paint, white sidewall tires and chrome rear fender skirts. The Economy Coach Company changed its name to the Memphis Coach Co. early in 1955.

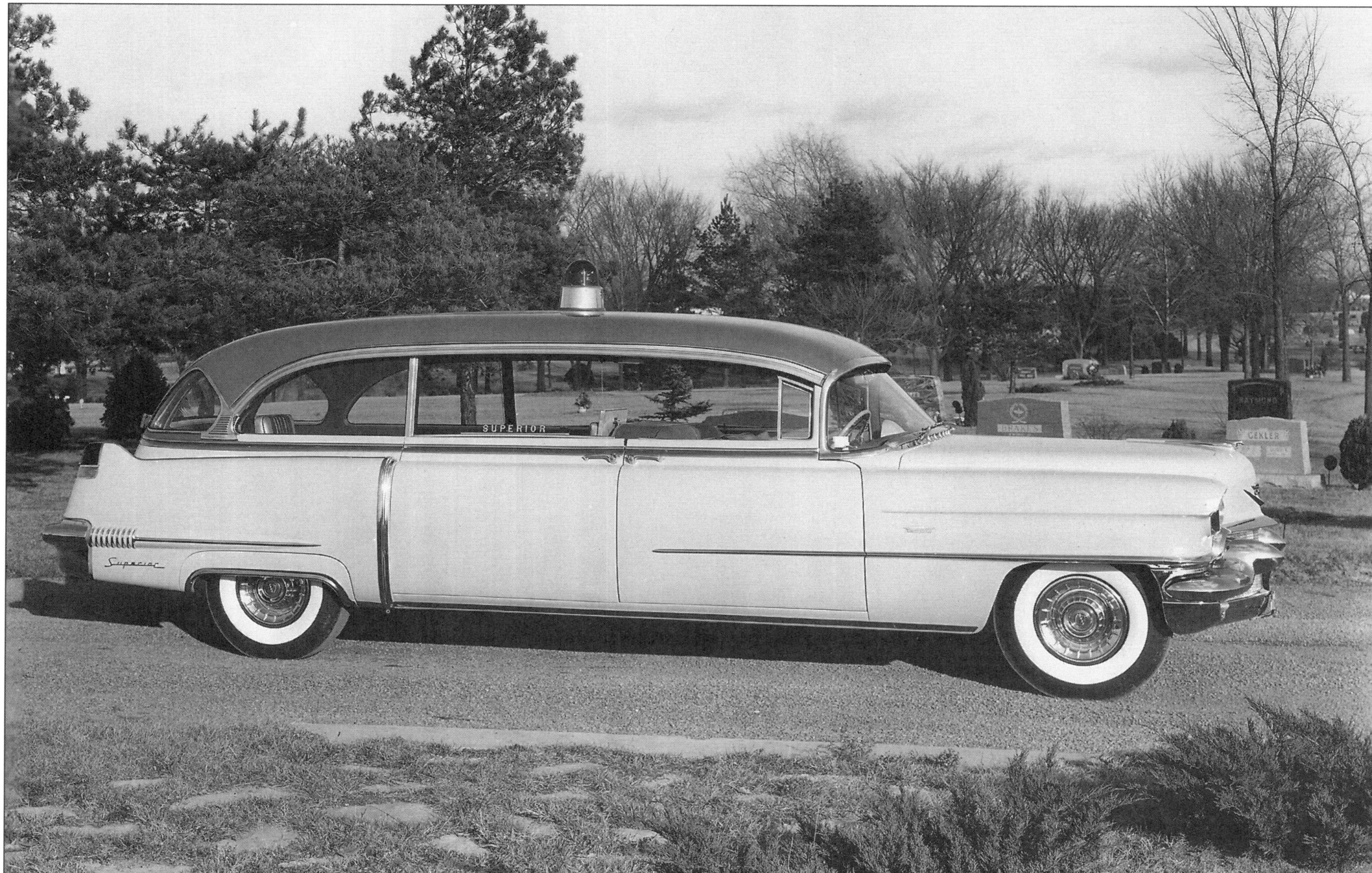

1956 SUPERIOR-CADILLAC BEAU MONDE COMBINATION - The Superior Coach Corp. introduced a series of stylish "pillarless hardtop" professional cars in 1955. The Superior-Cadillac Beau Monde models were available in Combination Funeral Car and Ambulance, Straight Funeral Coach and Floral Funeral Coach versions. This is the Combination Funeral Car/Ambulance. Note the vast open glass area and the folding attendant seat visible through the rear side window of this huge five-door hardtop.

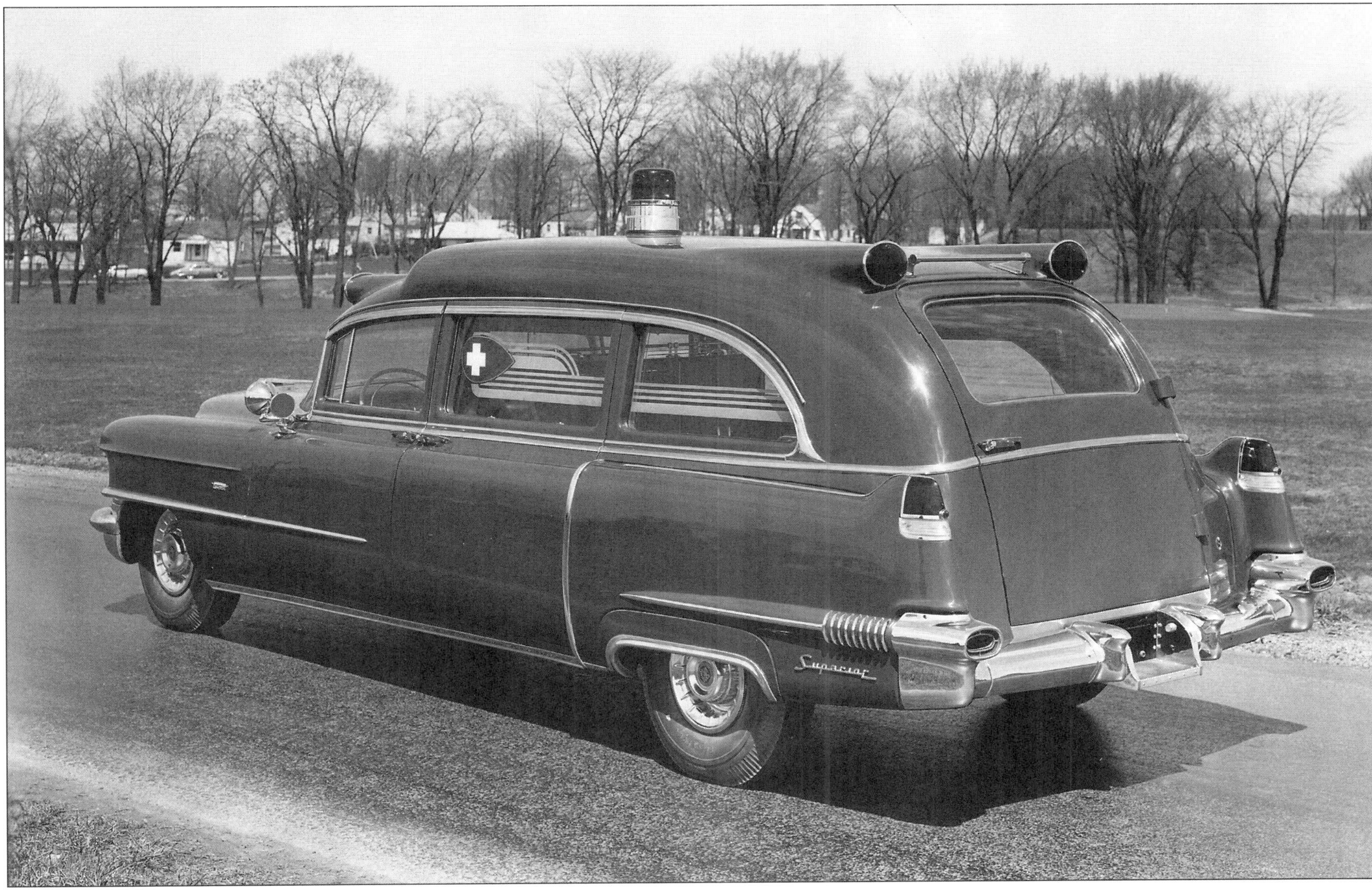

1956 SUPERIOR-CADILLAC SUPER RESCUER AMBULANCE - Superior's largest and most expensive ambulance was the high-headroom Super Rescuer on Cadillac commercial chassis. Designed for professional ambulance operators, rescue squads and fire departments, the Super Rescuer, with 51 inches of rear compartment headroom, could accommodate as many as four stretcher patients, plus two medical attendants. Note the rear bumper step, and large, oval rear roof lights.

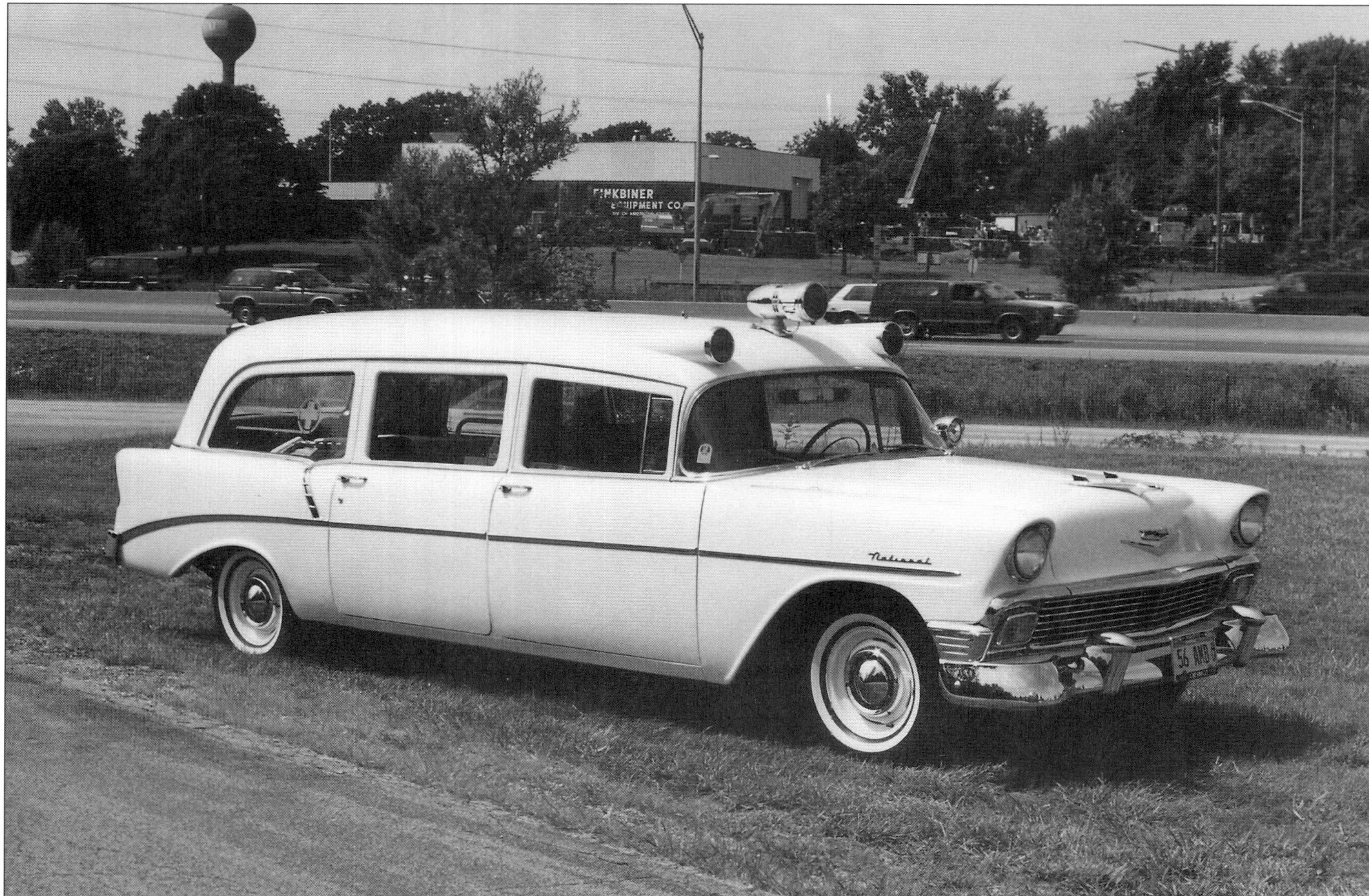

1956 NATIONAL-CHEVROLET MINUTEMAN AMBULANCE - The National Body Mfg. Co. of Knightstown, Indiana, produced ambulances and funeral cars on a wide range of chassis from 1948 into the 1960s. National did this straight ambulance conversion of a Chevrolet 210 in 1956. This fully restored 1956 National-Chevrolet Minuteman was among the participants at the 1998 Professional Car Society National Meet held in Burr Ridge, Illinois.

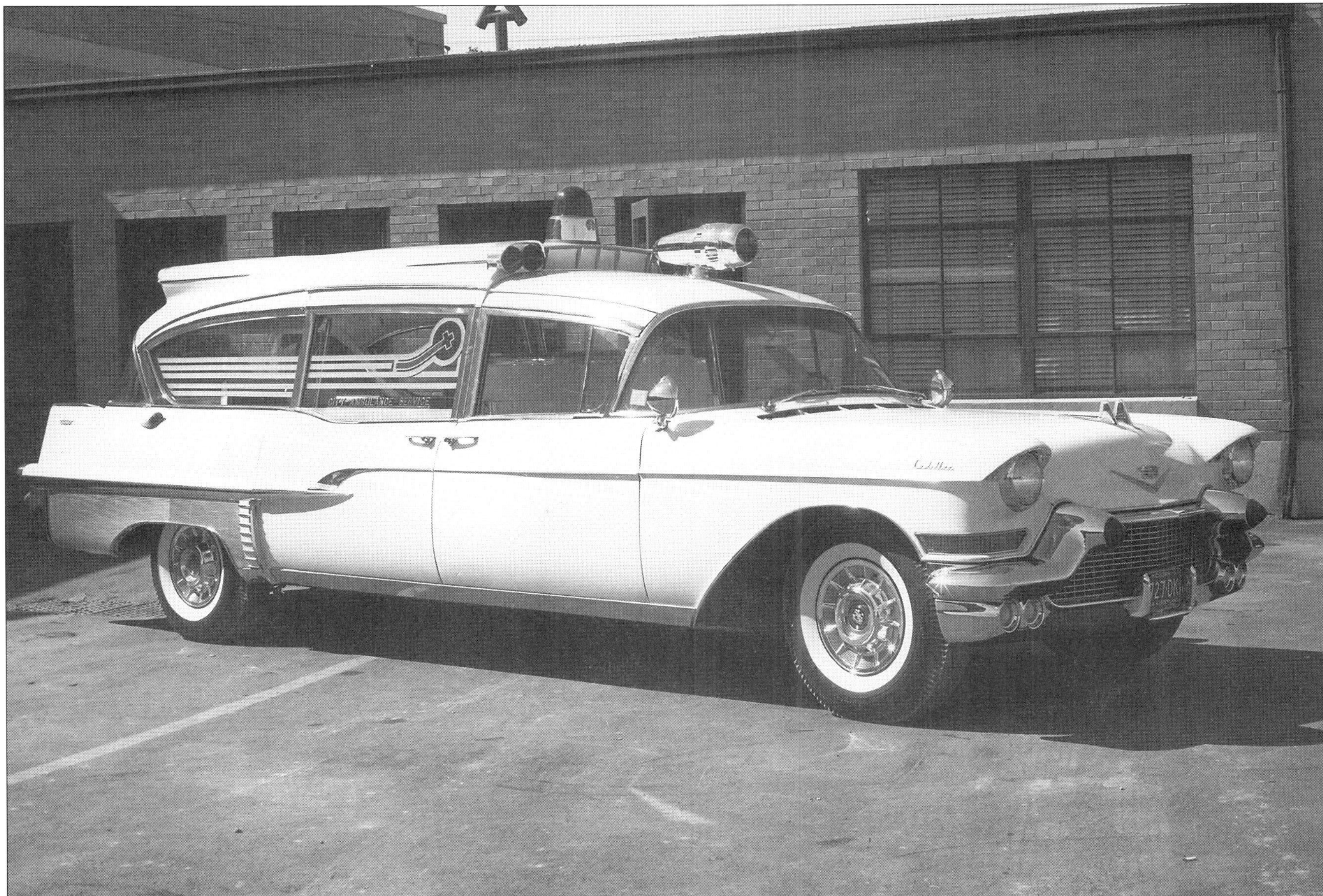

1957 SUPERIOR-CADILLAC RESCUER AMBULANCE - Superior Coach introduced all-new "Criterion" hardtop styling for its totally redesigned 1957 professional cars, including ambulances. This is the 1957 Superior-Cadillac Rescuer 48-inch Ambulance. Note the raised rear roof area and Cadillac Fleetwood-style lower rear quarter panel trim.

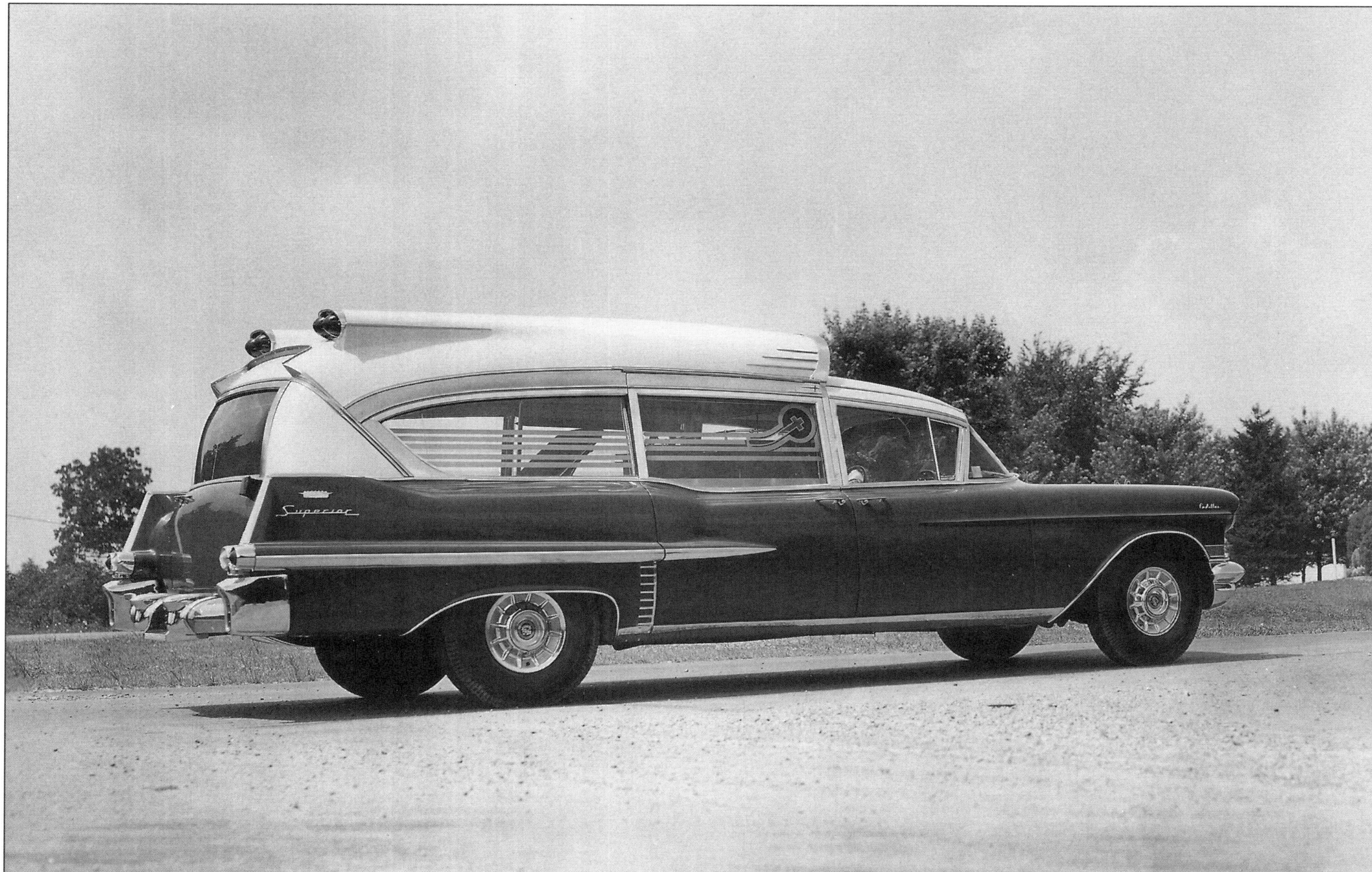

1957 SUPERIOR-CADILLAC SUPER RESCUER AMBULANCE - Superior Coach offered three Cadillac-chassised ambulances for 1957. This family included the 43-inch standard-headroom Beau Monde, the 48-inch Rescuer and the 52-inch Super Rescuer. All were built on the new 158-inch wheelbase "X"-frame Cadillac commercial chassis powered by Cadillac's 300 horsepower, 365 cubic-inch V-8 engine. The rear roof of this ambulance was one huge piece of molded fiberglass. Note the closed quarter windows.

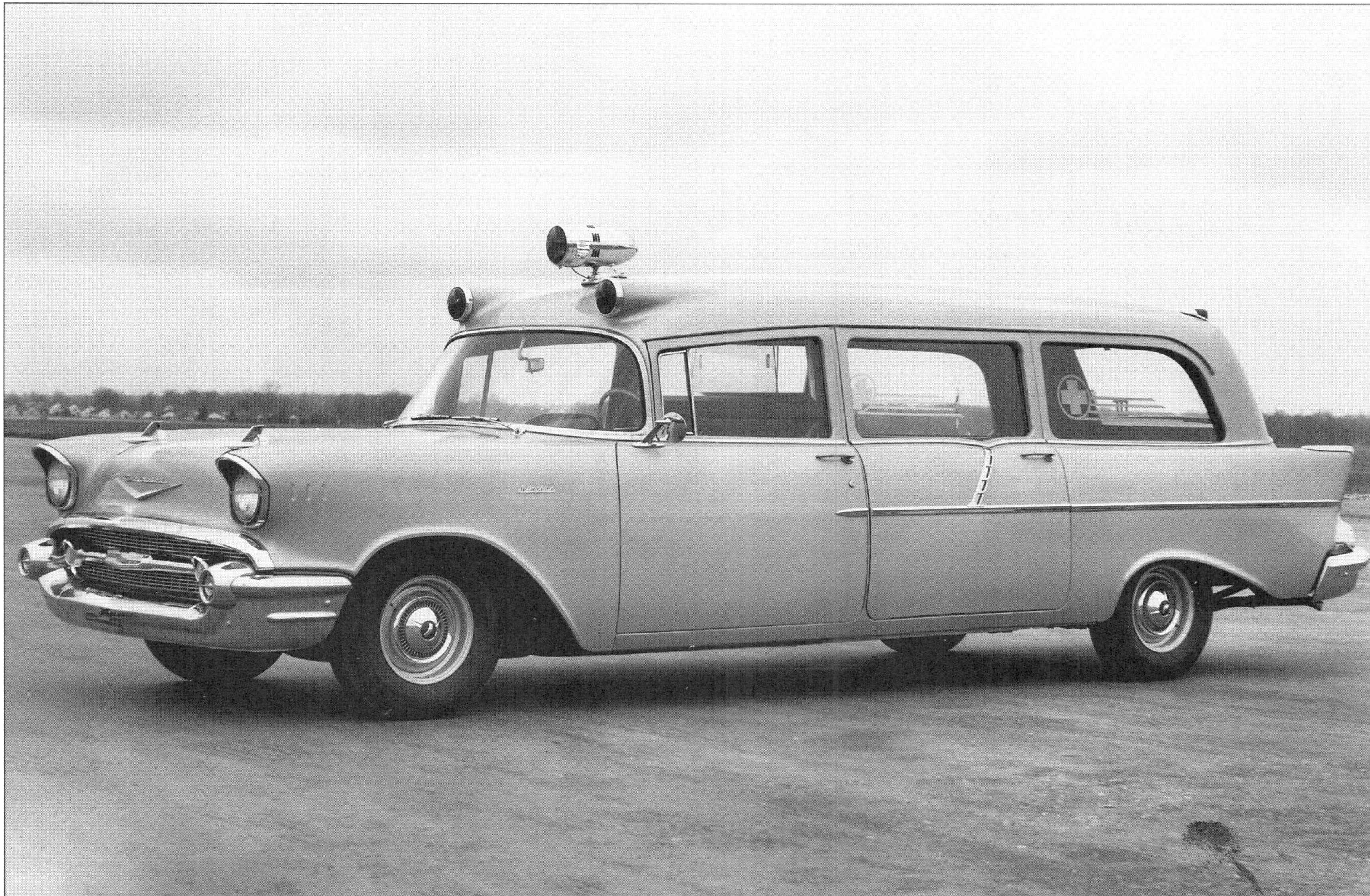

1957 MEMPHIAN-CHEVROLET AMBULANCE - The smaller, second-tier players in the ambulance manufacturing business during the fabulous fifties included the National Body Mfg. Co. of Knightstown, Indiana, Guy Barnette Co. of Memphis and the Memphis Coach Company. Memphis marketed its ambulances and hearses under the Memphian name. This is the 1957 Memphian-Chevrolet Long-Wheelbase Ambulance conversion of a Chevrolet 210.

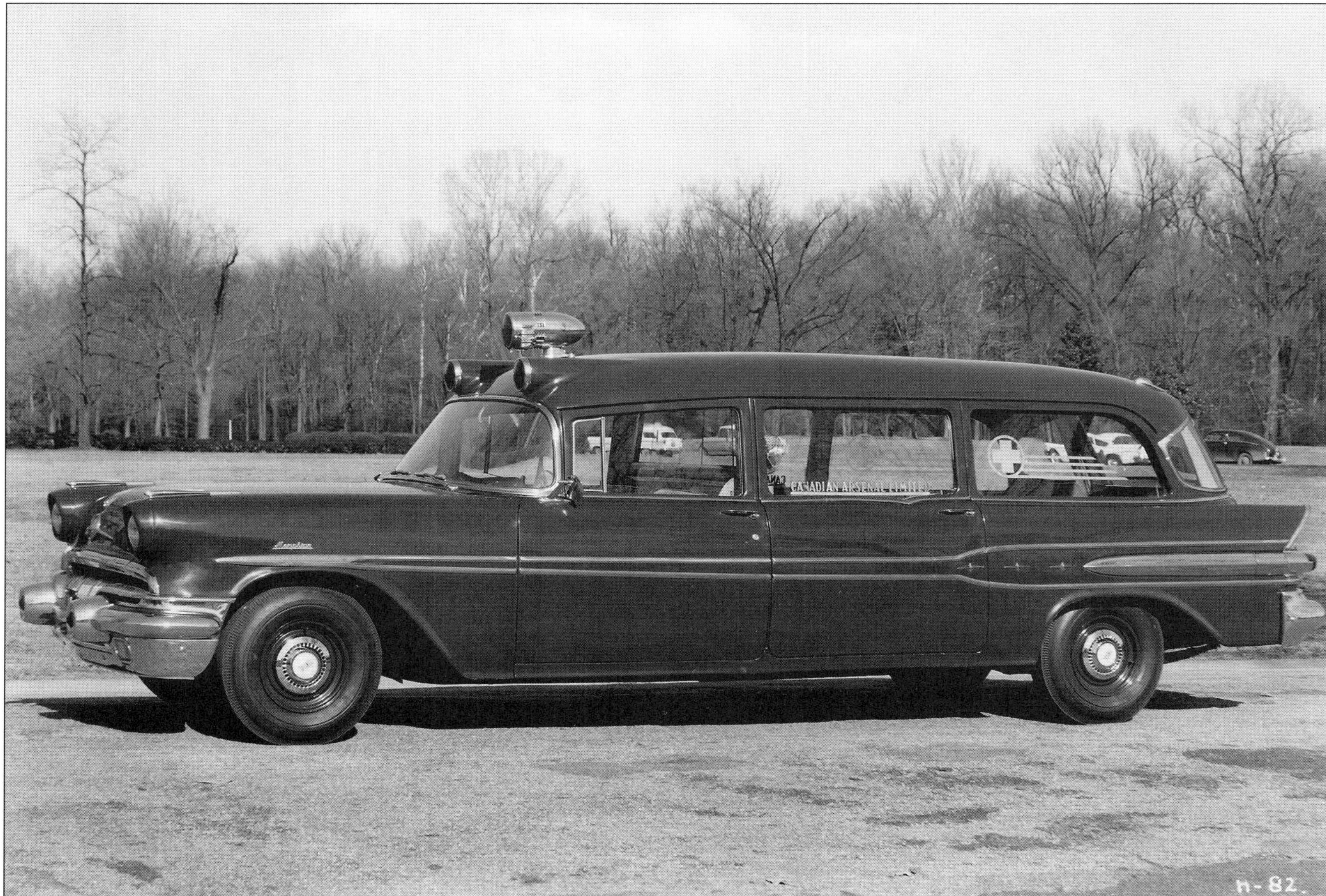

1957 MEMPHIAN-PONTIAC AMBULANCE - The Memphis Coach Co. built this 1957 Memphian-Pontiac Limousine Ambulance for the Canadian Arsenal Ltd. This vehicle survives in virtually original condition in a Canadian museum collection today. Note the small standard hubcaps and wraparound-type rear quarter windows.

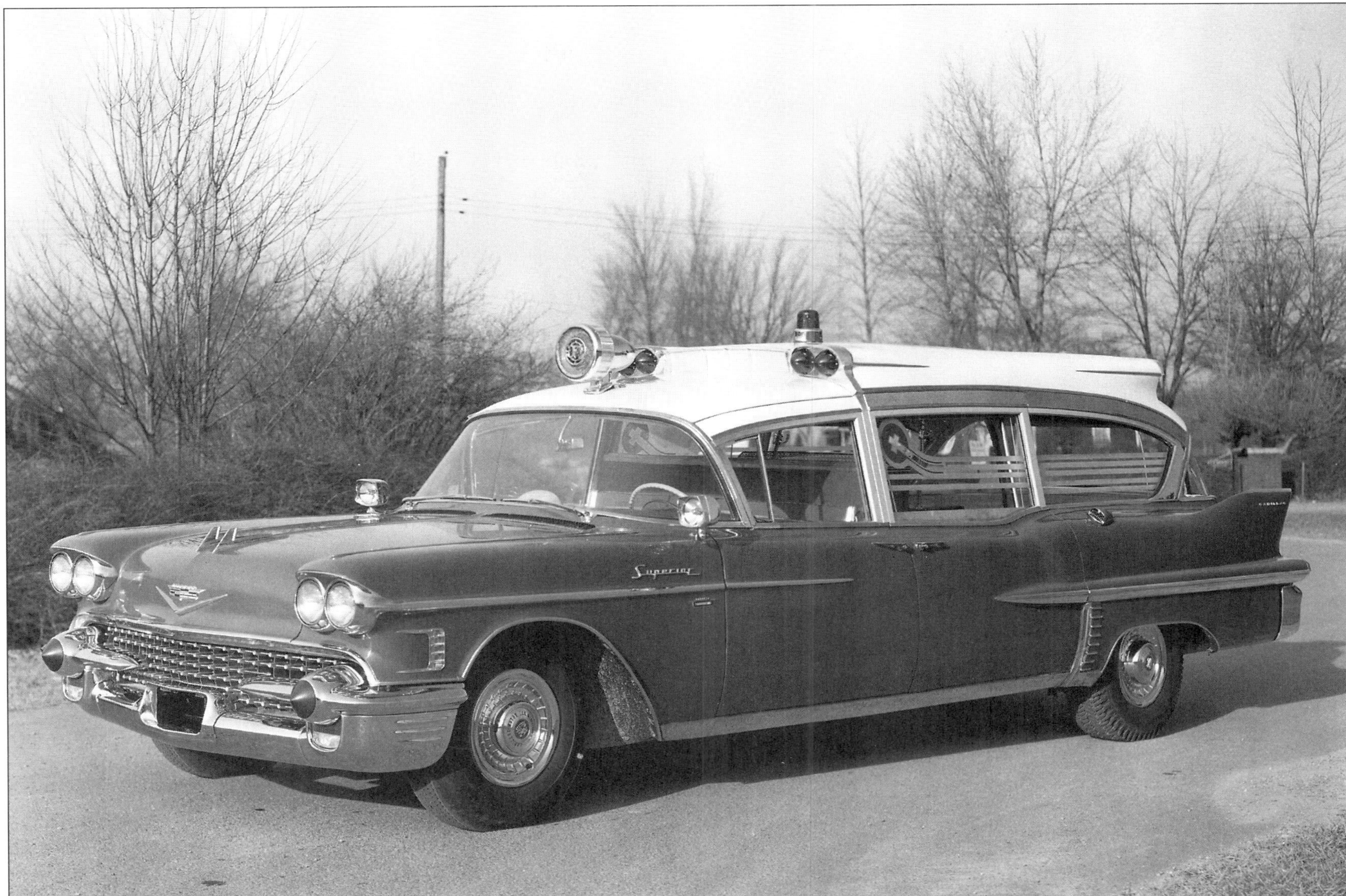

1958 SUPERIOR-CADILLAC RESCUER AMBULANCE - All American cars, including professional cars, were equipped with new dual headlight units for the 1958 model year. This is a 1958 Superior-Cadillac 48-inch Rescuer Ambulance. Warning equipment includes dual "bullet" red lights in the front of the raised rear roof and a big Federal "Q" coaster siren mounted above the windshield.

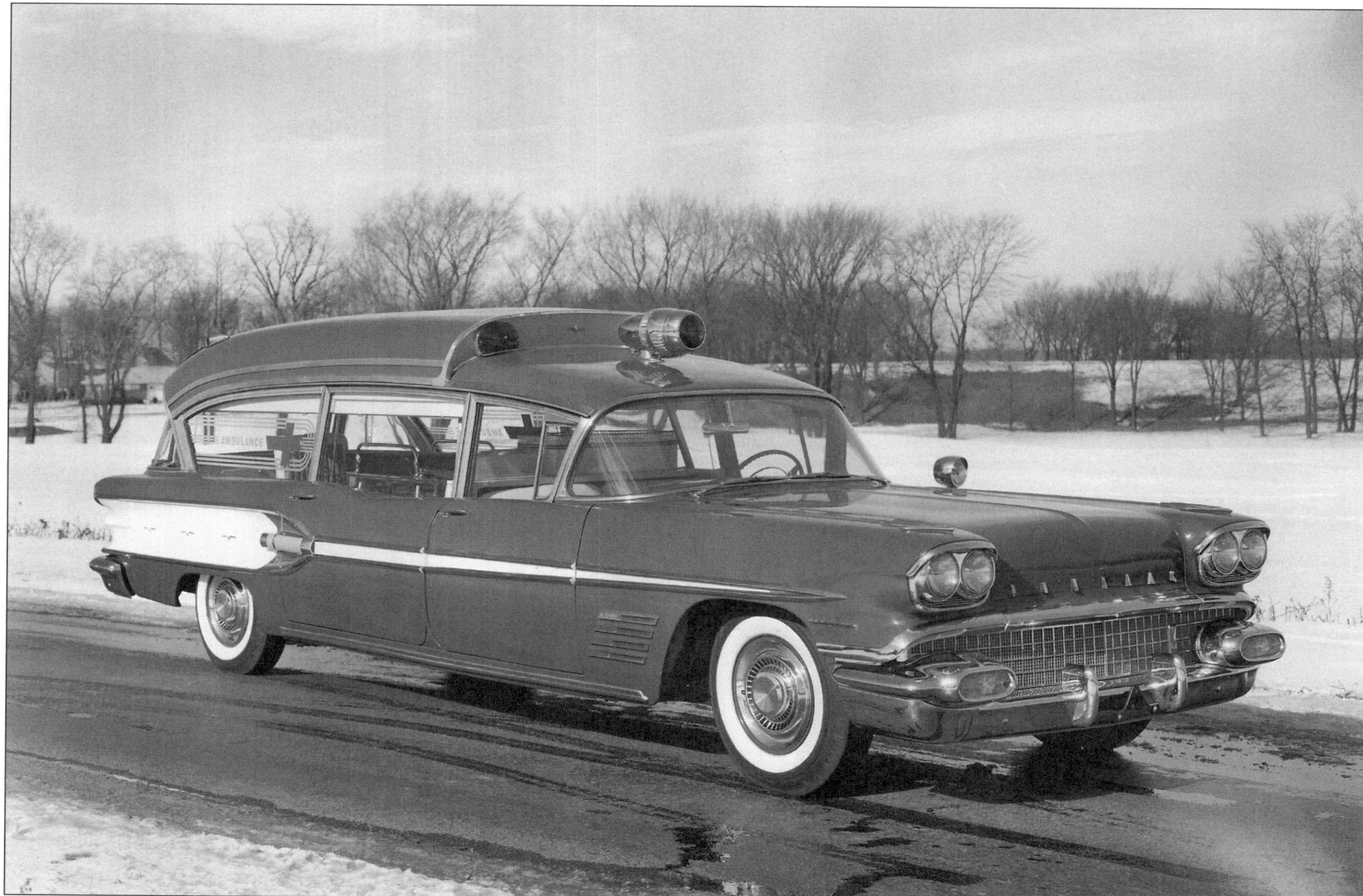

1958 SUPERIOR-PONTIAC CRITERION HIGHTOP AMBULANCE - Superior Coach offered its customers two distinct series of professional ambulances —three on the luxury Cadillac commercial chassis and two on less expensive stretched Pontiac Bonneville chassis. Both Superior-Pontiacs (the Criterion Crown with 42.5 inches of rear compartment headroom and the 46-inch Criterion Super Headroom version shown here) had step-type roofs.

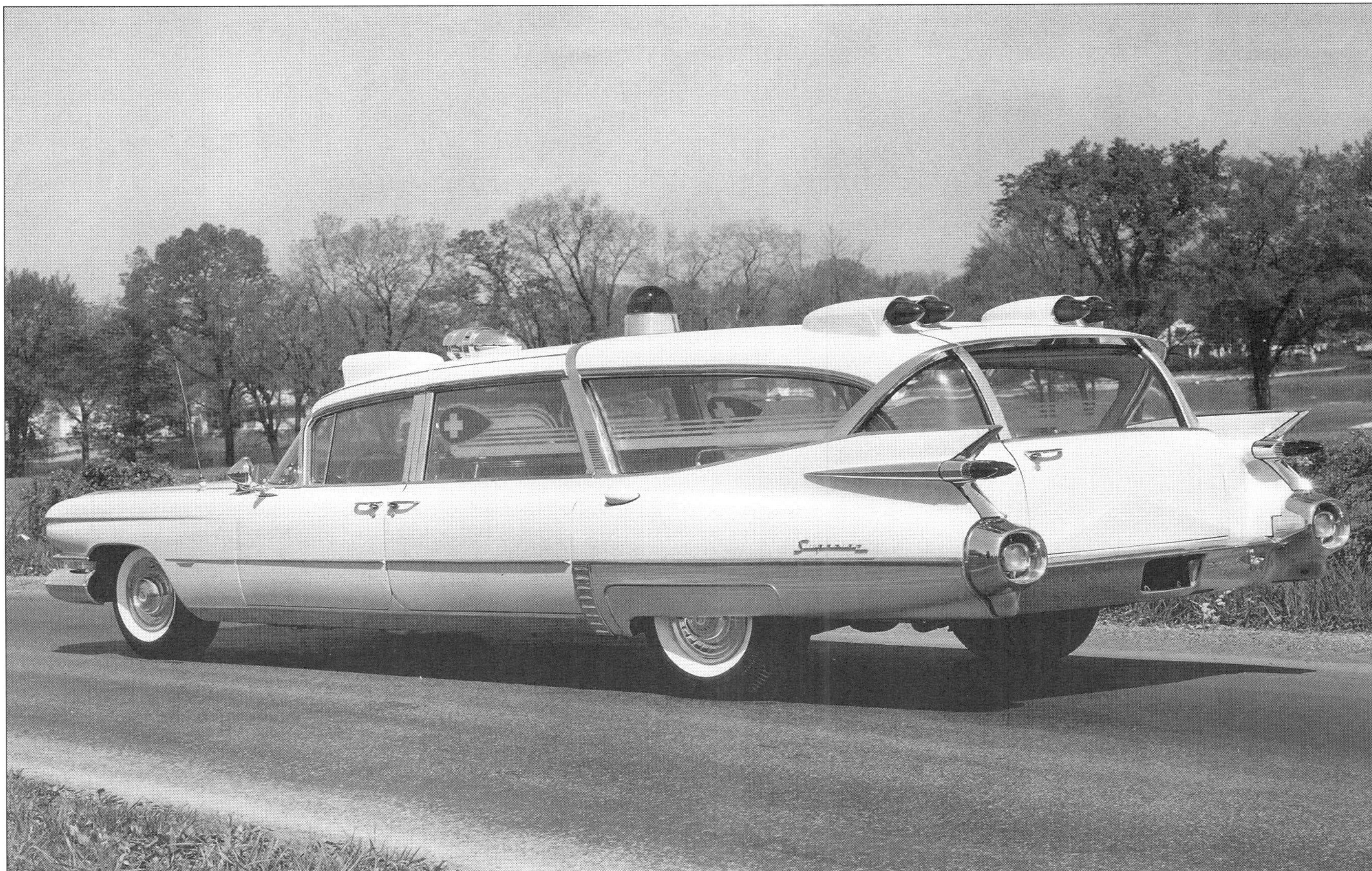

1959 SUPERIOR-CADILLAC CROWN ROYALE AMBULANCE - American passenger car styling reached its pinnacle of excess during the 1959 model year. Ambulance and funeral car stylists did their best to design dignified bodies for the flamboyant 1959 Cadillac commercial chassis with its soaring rocketship tailfins. Superior offered 1959 Cadillac ambulances in two series: Royale and Crown Royale. This is the Crown Royale 42-inch Limousine Ambulance with "up-and-over" C-pillar roof molding and extruded aluminum lower rear quarter panel trim.

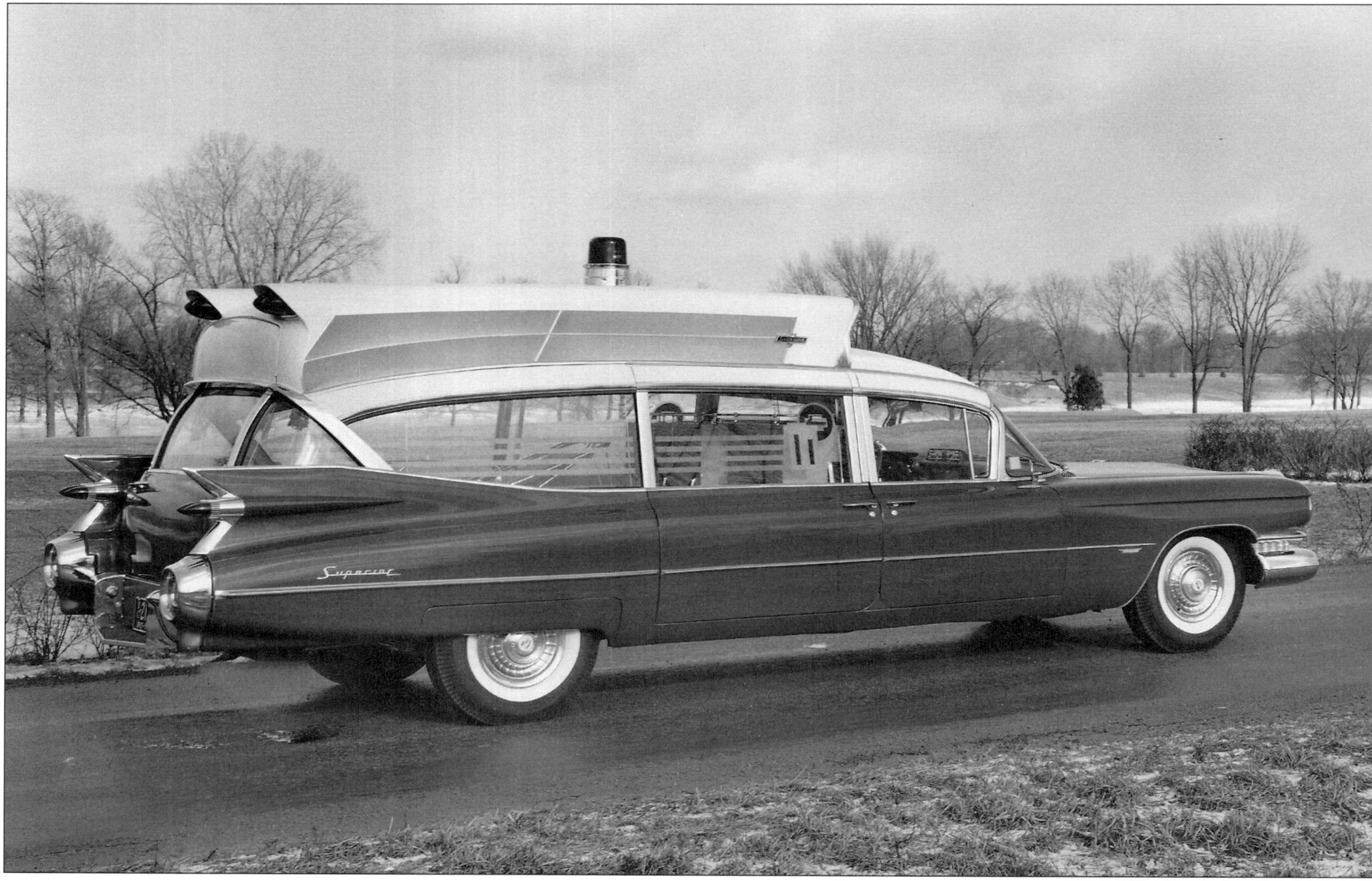

1959 SUPERIOR-CADILLAC ROYALE SUPER RESCUER - For 1959, Superior offered no fewer than *four* rear compartment headroom heights in its Cadillac ambulances in two series: Royale and the premium Crown Royale. The base model was the Royale with standard 42-inch headroom. The Crown Royale offered 43 inches. The raised-roof Royale Rescuer had 48 inches of interior working height while the top-line Royale Super Rescuer shown here boasted 54 inches of rear compartment headroom.

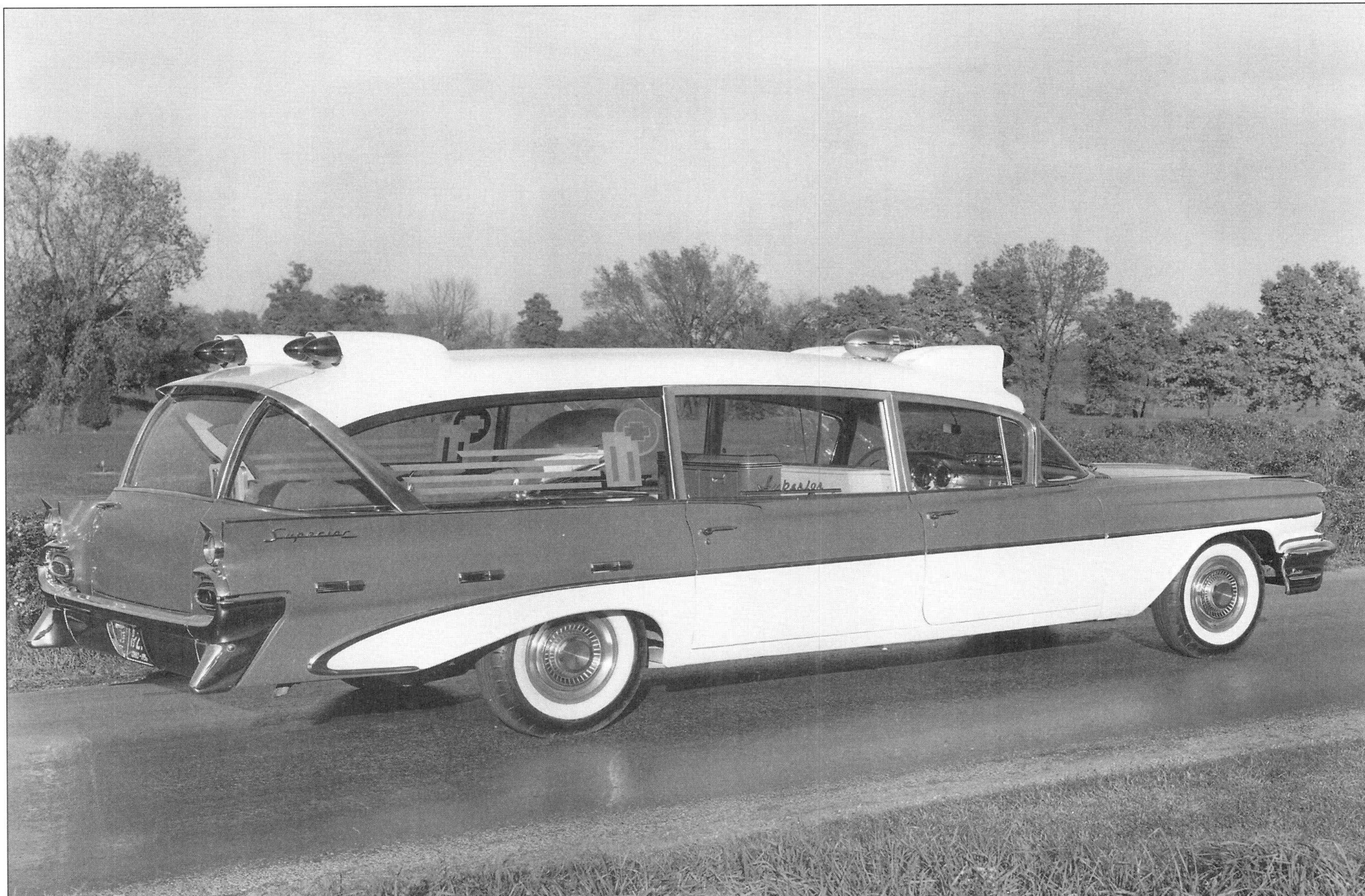

1959 SUPERIOR-PONTIAC CRITERION - Superior Coach offered two ambulances on the new Pontiac Wide-Track chassis for 1959. The standard headroom model was the 40.5-inch Superior-Pontiac Criterion shown here. The 1959 Pontiac's sweeping chrome side trim made a natural color break for two-toning, as exemplified on this extremely attractive white-and-red Criterion.

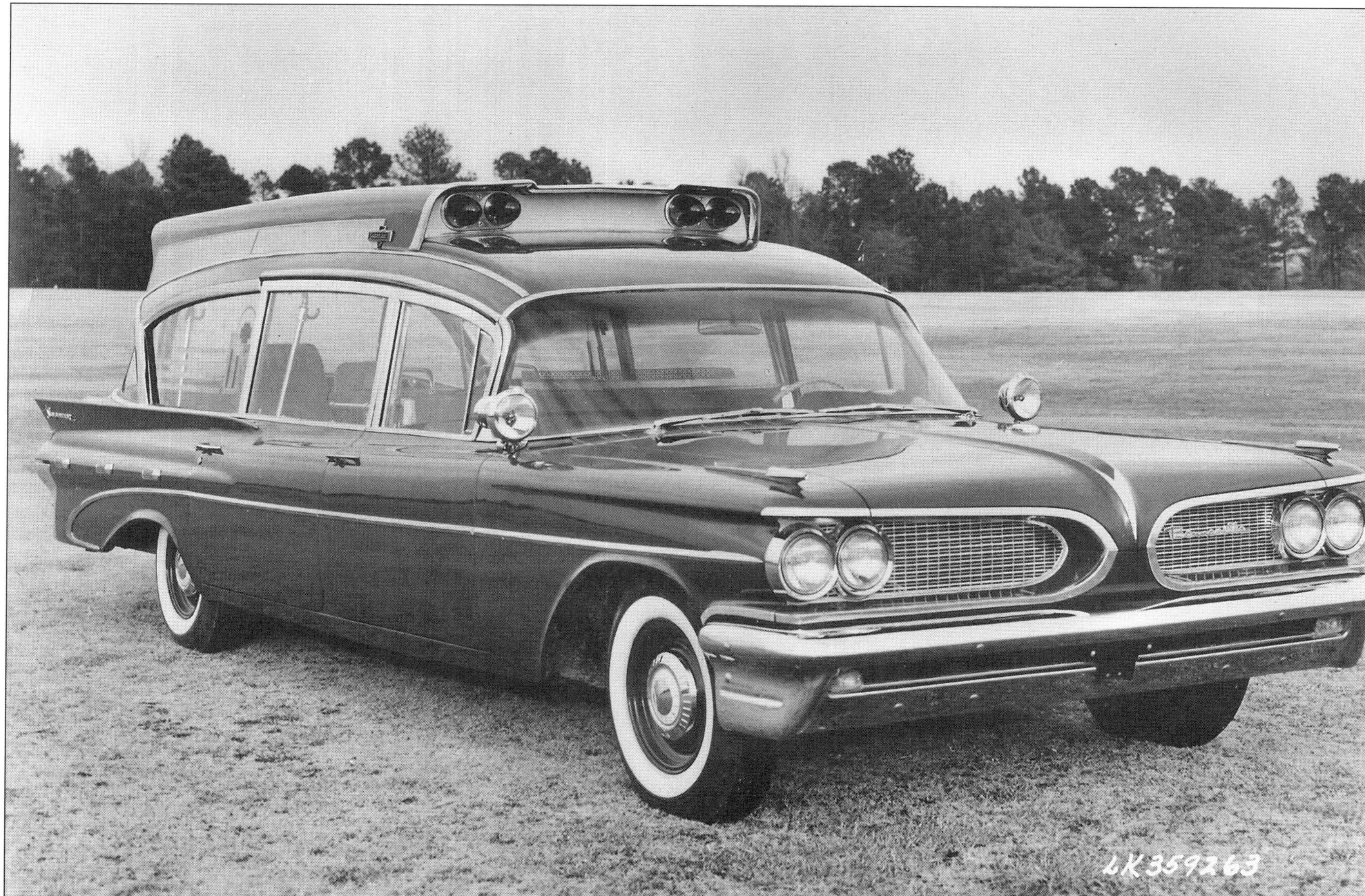

1959 SUPERIOR-PONTIAC CRITERION SUBURBAN HIGHTOP AMBULANCE - The 1959 Superior-Pontiacs were built on a stretched Bonneville chassis with a 148-inch wheelbase. The top model in the 1959 Superior-Pontiac ambulance lineup was the Criterion Suburban which offered 46 inches of rear compartment headroom. Note the raised rear roof, dual remote-control spotlights and standard small hubcaps.

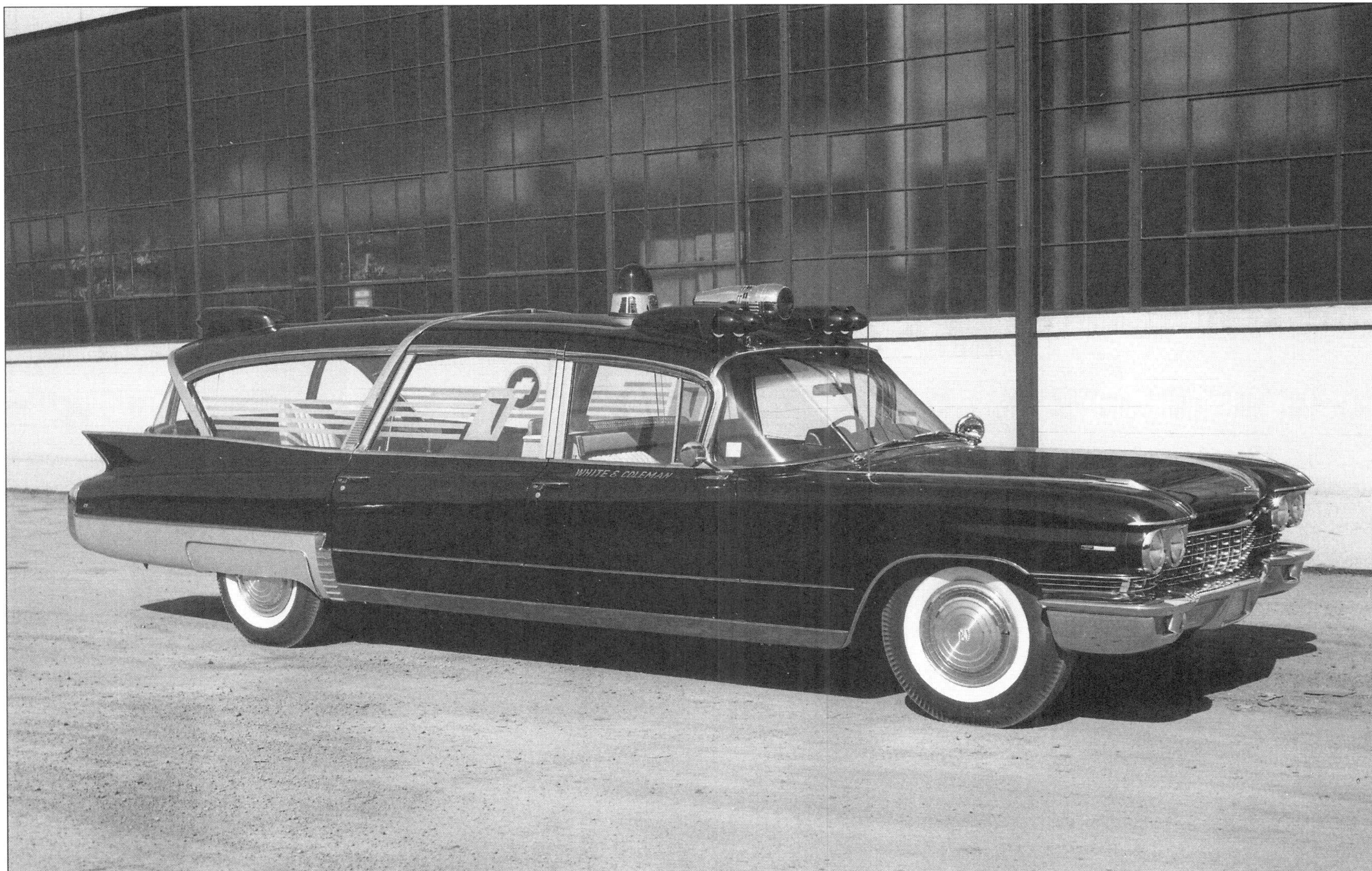

1960 SUPERIOR-CADILLAC CROWN ROYALE AMBULANCE - The 1960 Cadillac commercial chassis showed the same welcome styling restraint as Cadillac's 1960 passenger cars, with subdued tailfins and a lot less chrome. Superior again offered three ambulance headroom heights in two series, Royale and Crown Royale. This is the 1960 Superior-Cadillac Crown Royale Limousine Ambulance with 43 inches of rear compartment headroom and extruded aluminum lower quarter panel trim.

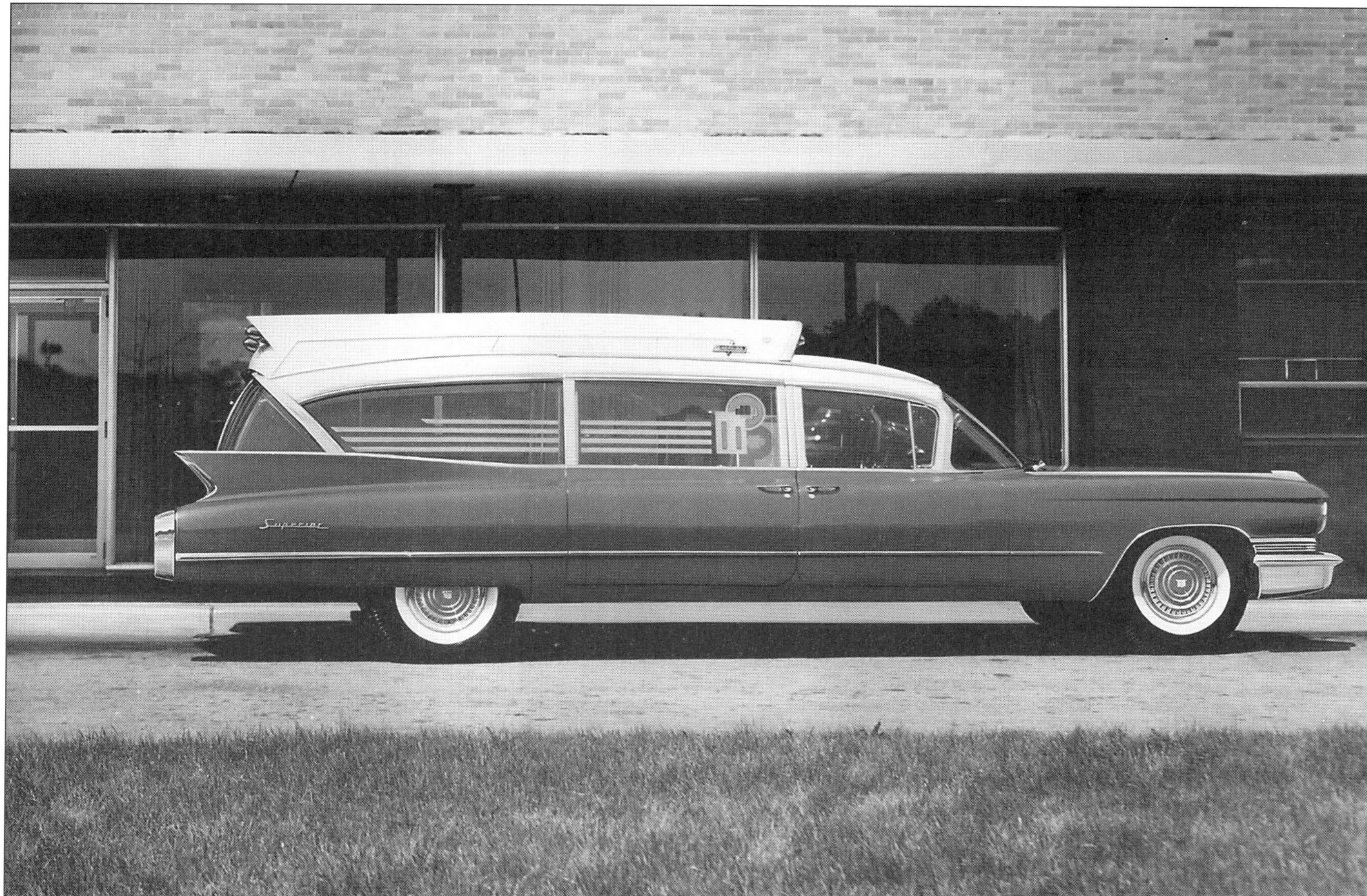

1960 SUPERIOR-CADILLAC ROYALE SUPER RESCUER - Parked outside a Lima, Ohio, hospital for the company photographer, this 1960 Superior-Cadillac Royale Super Rescuer Ambulance has no warning lights except for the bullet-type red flashers at the front and rear of its raised rear roof. Some operators preferred to install their own sirens, lights, etc. after delivery. White-over-red remained the most popular exterior color choice for ambulances.

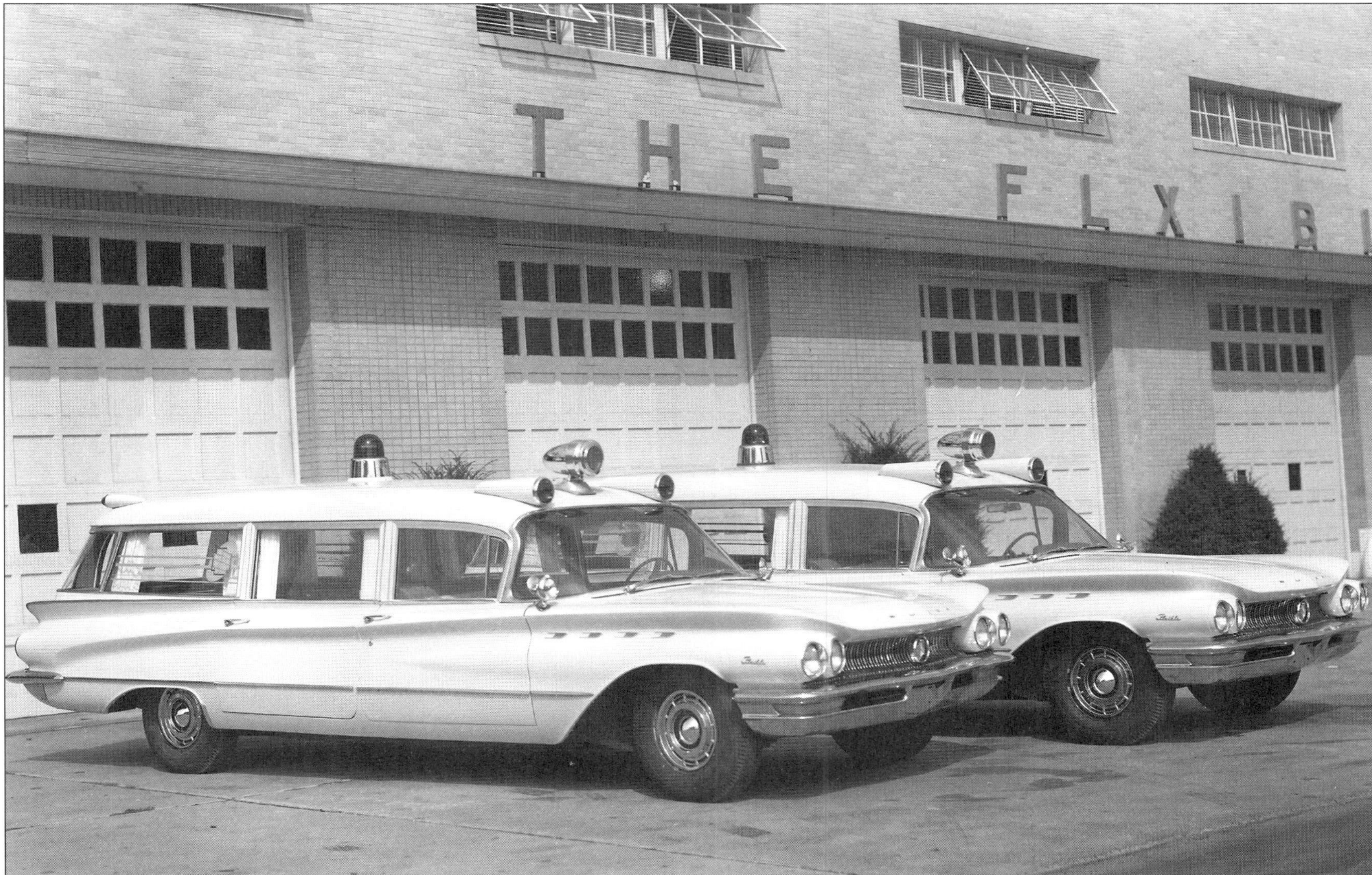

1960 FLXIBLE-BUICK PREMIER AMBULANCES - After a six-year hiatus, the Flxible company of Loudonville, Ohio, resumed ambulance and funeral car production in 1959, again using Buick chassis exclusively. This matched pair of 1960 Flxible-Buick Premier Ambulances was photographed outside the Flxible plant prior to delivery to a fleet customer. Note the "airline" type sliding window drapes, tunnel lights fore and aft and Federal Beacon Ray mounted in the center of the roof.

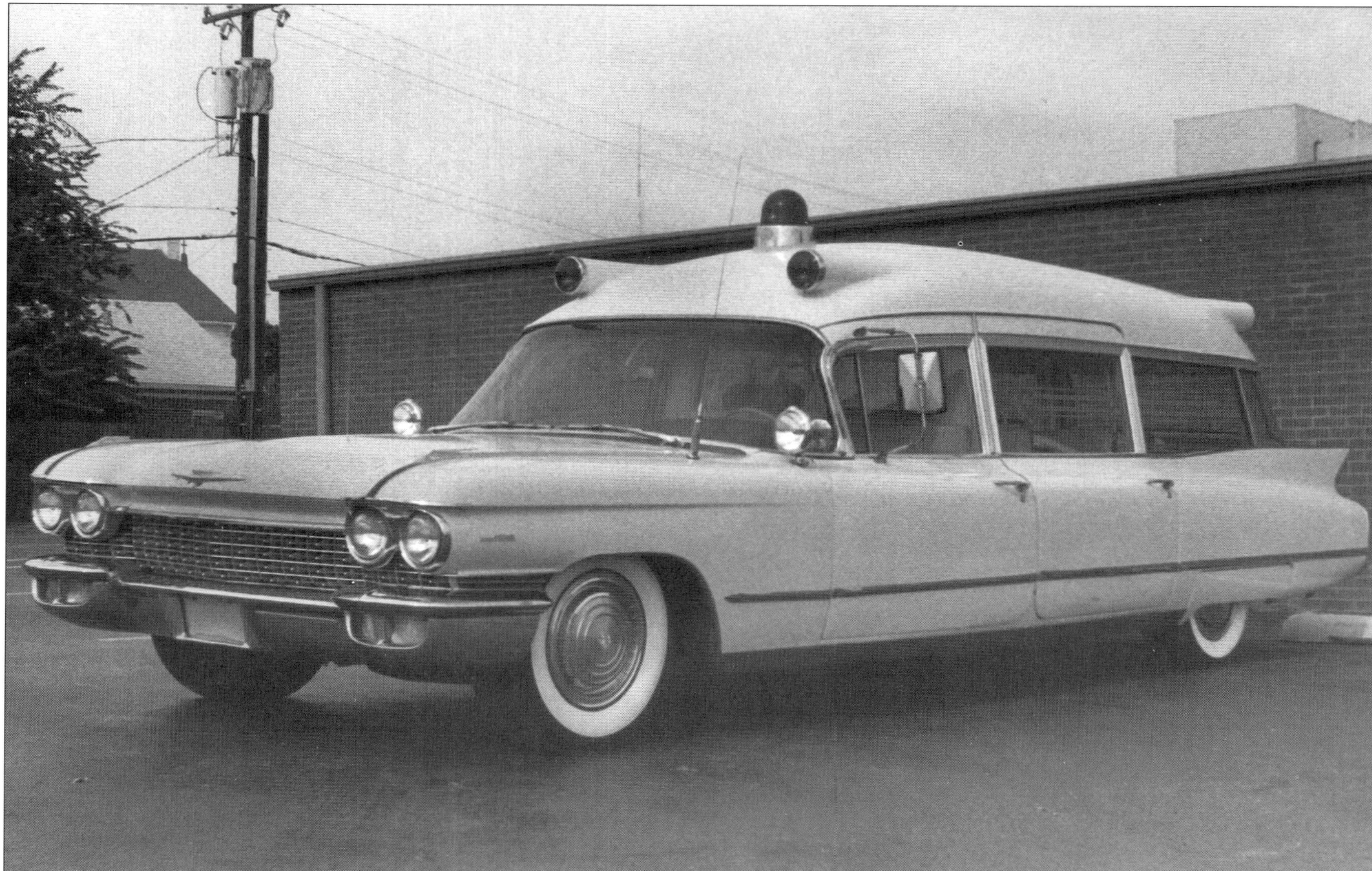

1960 MILLER-METEOR CADILLAC "VOLUNTEER" AMBULANCE - In 1956 the Meteor Motor Car Company of Piqua, Ohio, and the A. J. Miller Company of Bellefontaine, Ohio, merged to form the Miller-Meteor Division of Wayne Corp. Miller-Meteor Cadillac ambulances were built in the former A. J. Miller plant in Bellefontaine from 1957 through the 1960 model year, when production was transferred to the former Meteor plant in Piqua. This is a 1960 Miller-Meteor Cadillac Volunteer Hightop Ambulance owned by Steven B. Loftin of Tulsa, Oklahoma.

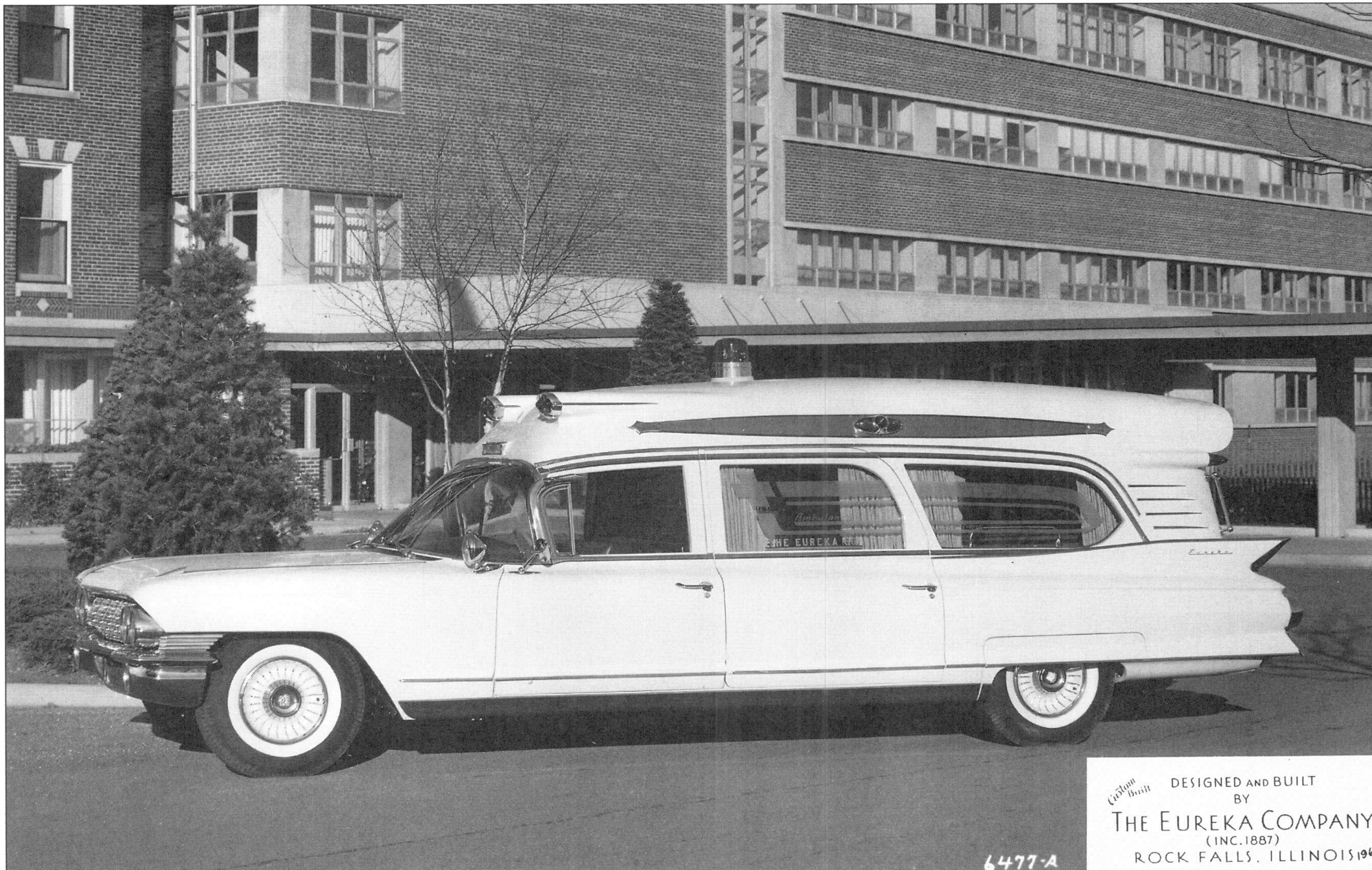

1961 EUREKA-CADILLAC HI-BOY AMBULANCE - The Eureka Company's premium hightop Cadillac ambulance was called the Eureka Hi-Boy. Interior appointments included a full-width, hand-rubbed, solid maple medicine cabinet, ample storage for a resuscitator, oxygen and other emergency equipment and carrying capacity for four patients. Note the color-keyed Cadillac wheel covers and the grab handles built into the rear of the curved, overhanging rear roof.

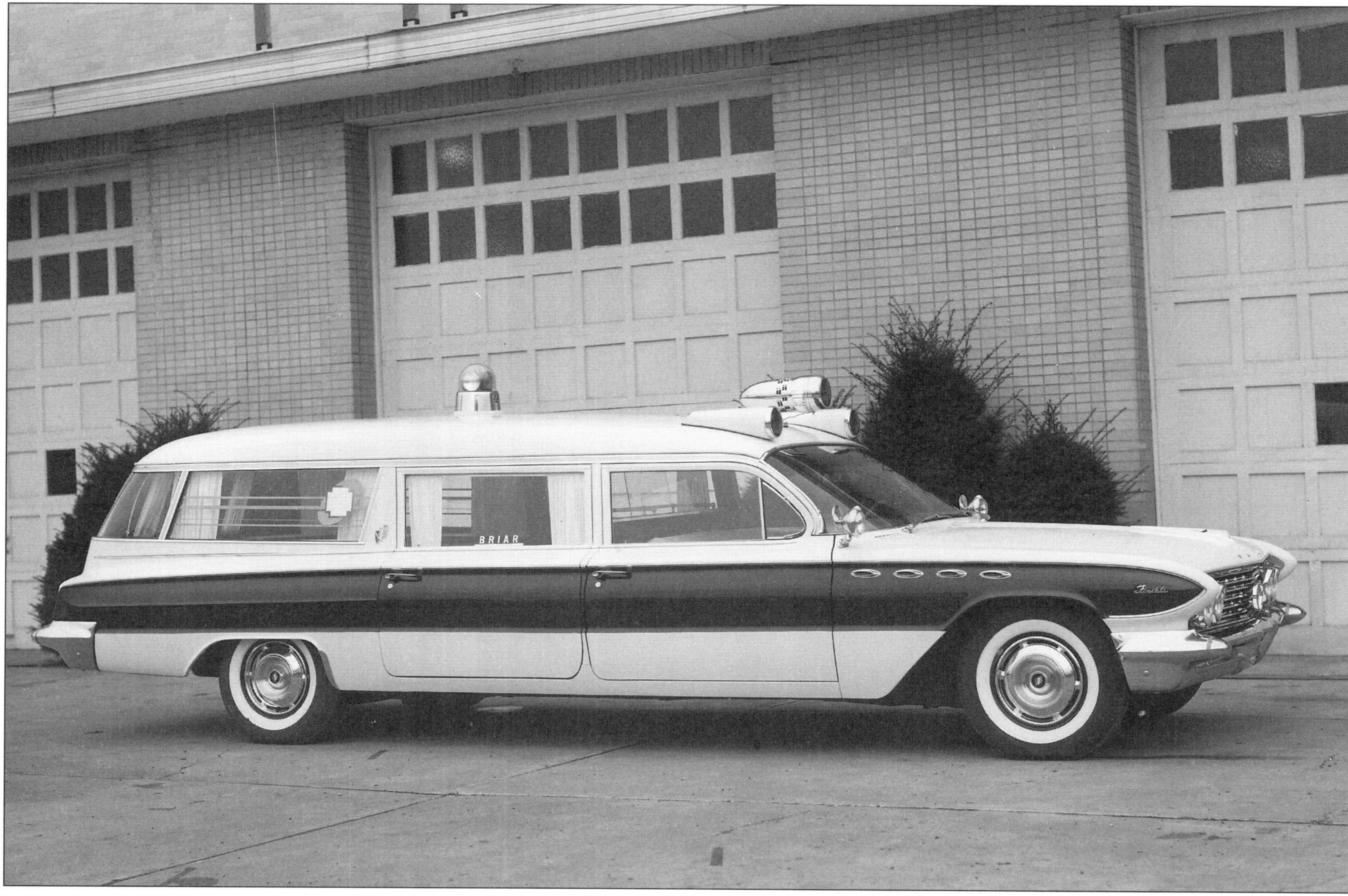

1961 FLXIBLE-BUICK PREMIER AMBULANCE - The 1961 Flxible-Buick Premier was an uncommonly handsome emergency vehicle. The 1961 Buick's pointed front fenders, full-length body character lines, and the long, low Flxible roofline make this classic limousine-style ambulance look longer than it actually was. Note the roof tunnel lights and the Federal coaster siren mounted on the roof.

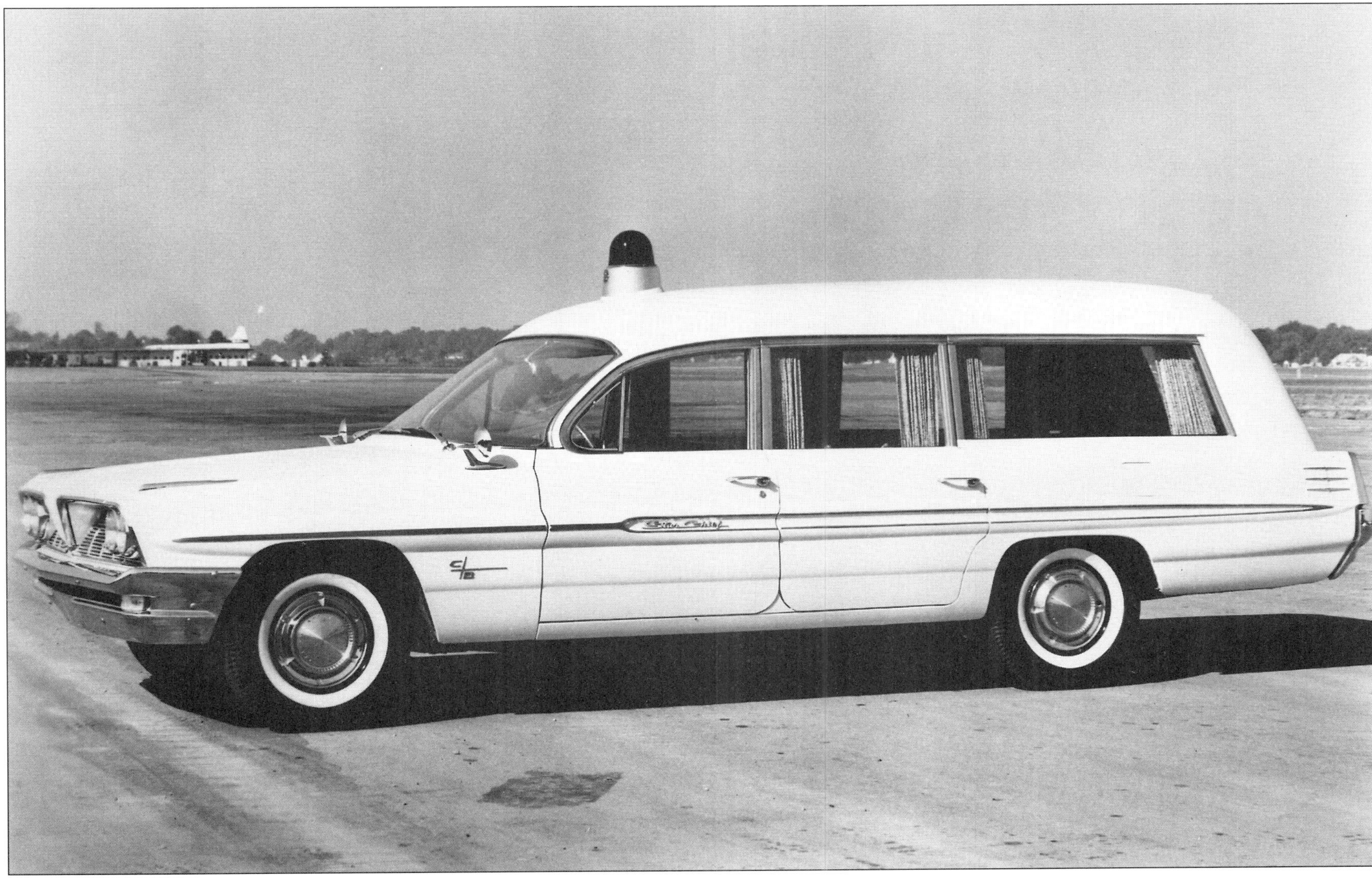

1961 COTNER/BEVINGTON PONTIAC COMBINATION - In 1959 the Comet Coach Co. of Blytheville, Arkansas, sold the Comet name to the Ford Motor Company to use on a new line of Mercury compacts. For 1960, the company adopted the names of its two owners and became the Cotner/Bevington Corp. Comet and Cotner/Bevington built most of their ambulances, funeral coaches and limousines on Oldsmobile chassis, but C/B built some Pontiacs, too. This standard-wheelbase, raised-roof combination is something of a rarity.

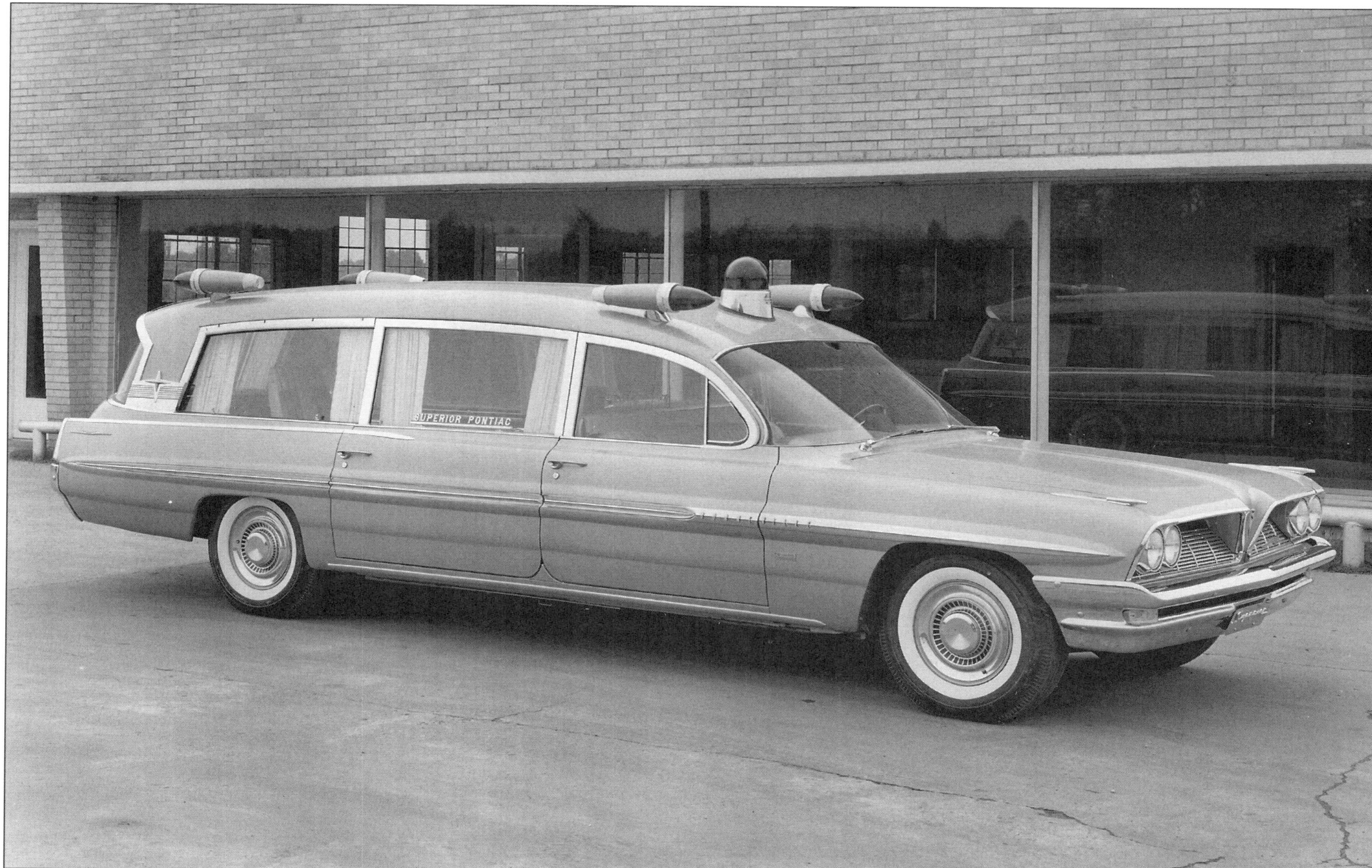

1961 SUPERIOR-PONTIAC CRITERION AMBULANCE - Posed outside Superior's Southern Division showroom in Kosiusko, Mississippi, is this spanking new 1961 Superior-Pontiac Criterion Ambulance. Note the bullet-type red warning lights front and rear and the Beacon Ray mounted above the windshield. The Criterion was Superior's standard headroom (40.5-inch) Pontiac ambulance. The raised-roof Criterion 46-inch Super Headroom Pontiac Ambulance was also still available.

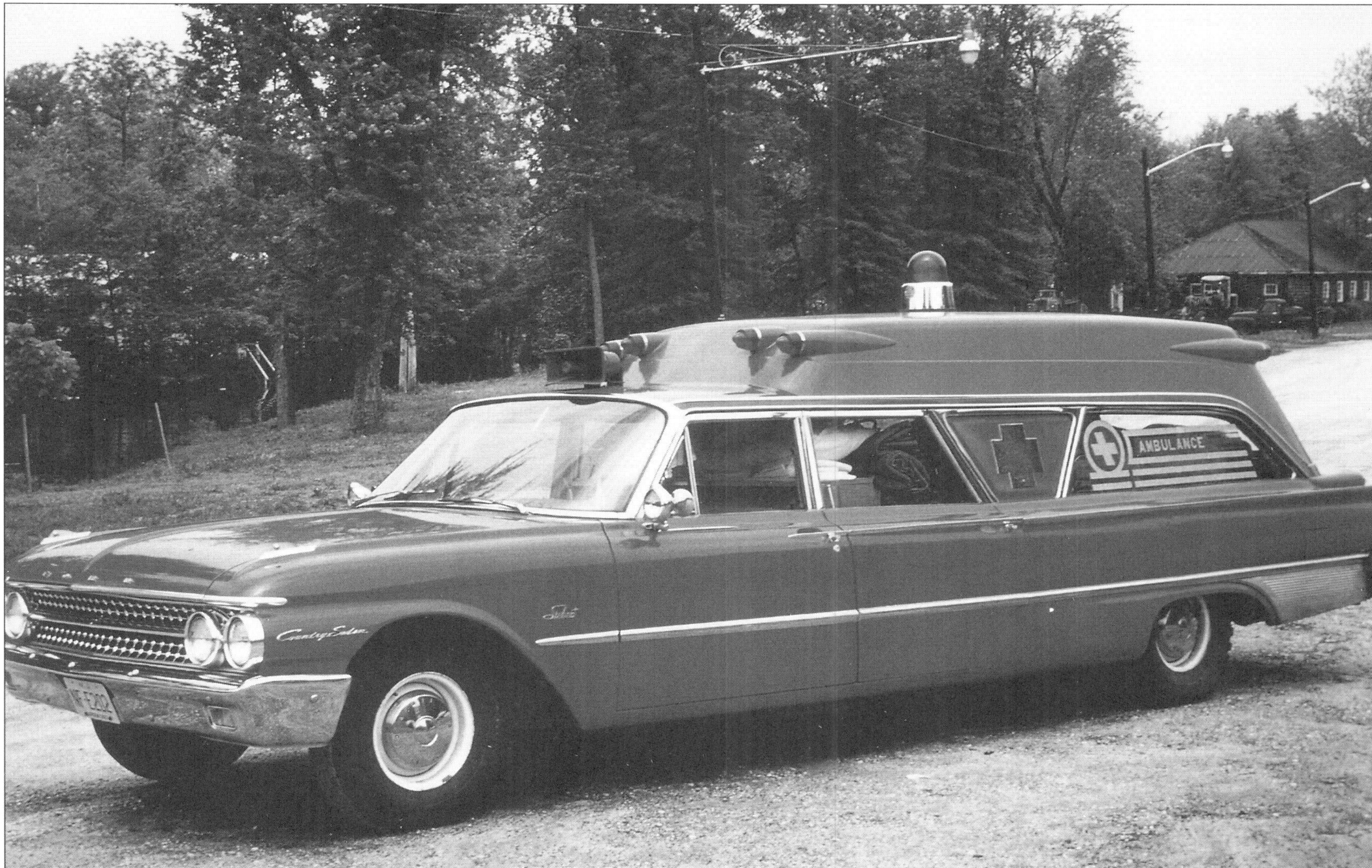

1961 SIEBERT-FORD ARISTOCRAT AMBULANCE - The Shop of Siebert Associates of Toledo and Waterville, Ohio, specialized in funeral coach, ambulance and limousine conversions of standard Ford passenger cars from 1933 through 1956. Siebert resumed professional car production from 1960-1964. Siebert's top-line, long-wheelbase ambulance and hearse conversions were called Siebert Aristocrats. The basis for this high-headroom ambulance conversion was a 1961 Ford Country Sedan station wagon.

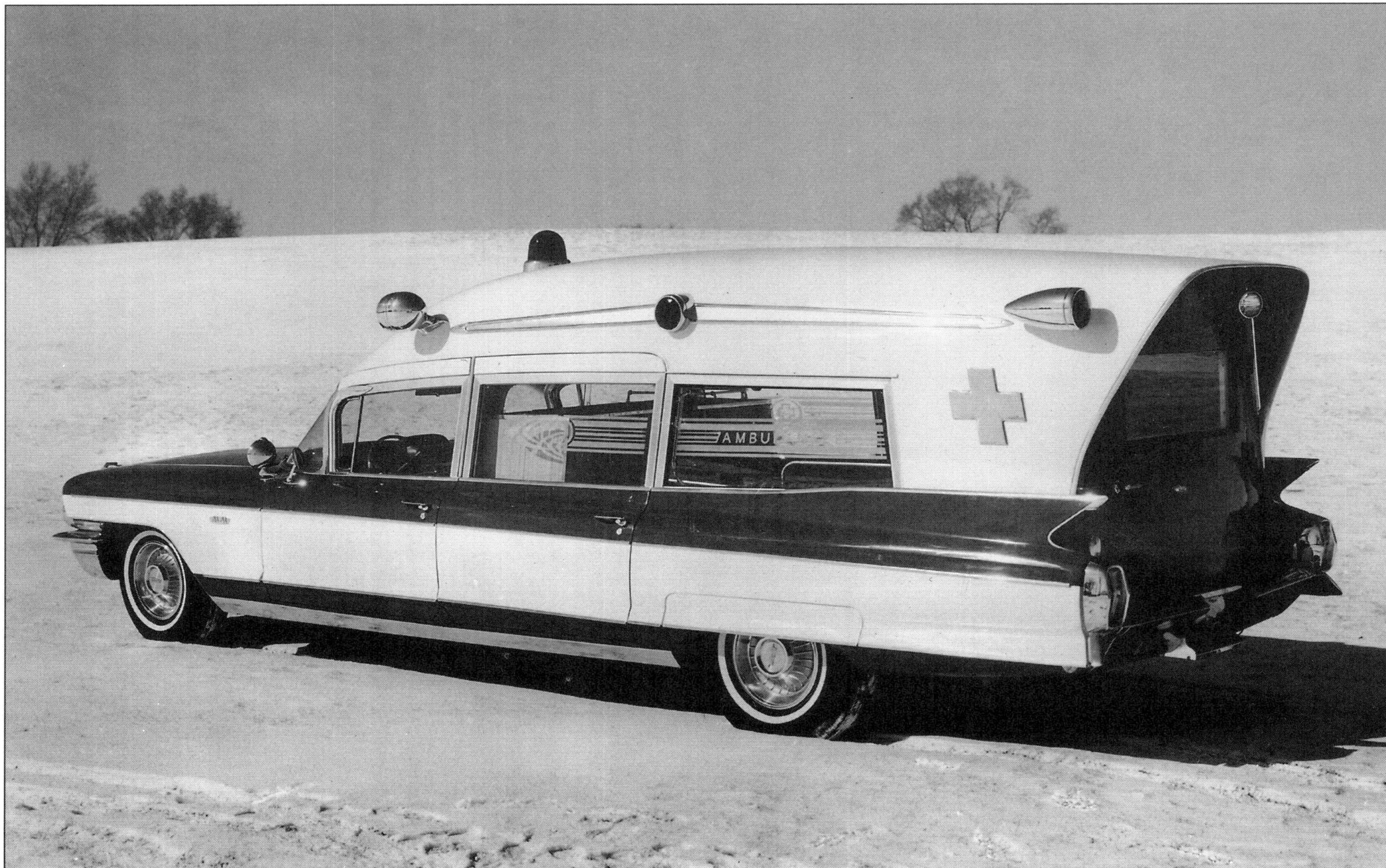

1962 MILLER-METEOR CADILLAC GUARDIAN AMBULANCE - One of the most unique ambulances ever seen in the U.S. was Miller-Meteor's Guardian, which was built for only three model years: 1960, 1961 and 1962. The ultrahigh-headroom Guardian was designed for heavy rescue service by rescue squads, fire departments, civil defense units and other agencies involved in disaster work. The Guardian's roof extended rearward, forming a protective canopy over the rear loading door area, with 52 inches of headroom. It is not known how many of these heavy-duty rescue vehicles Miller-Meteor built during the Guardian's three-year production run.

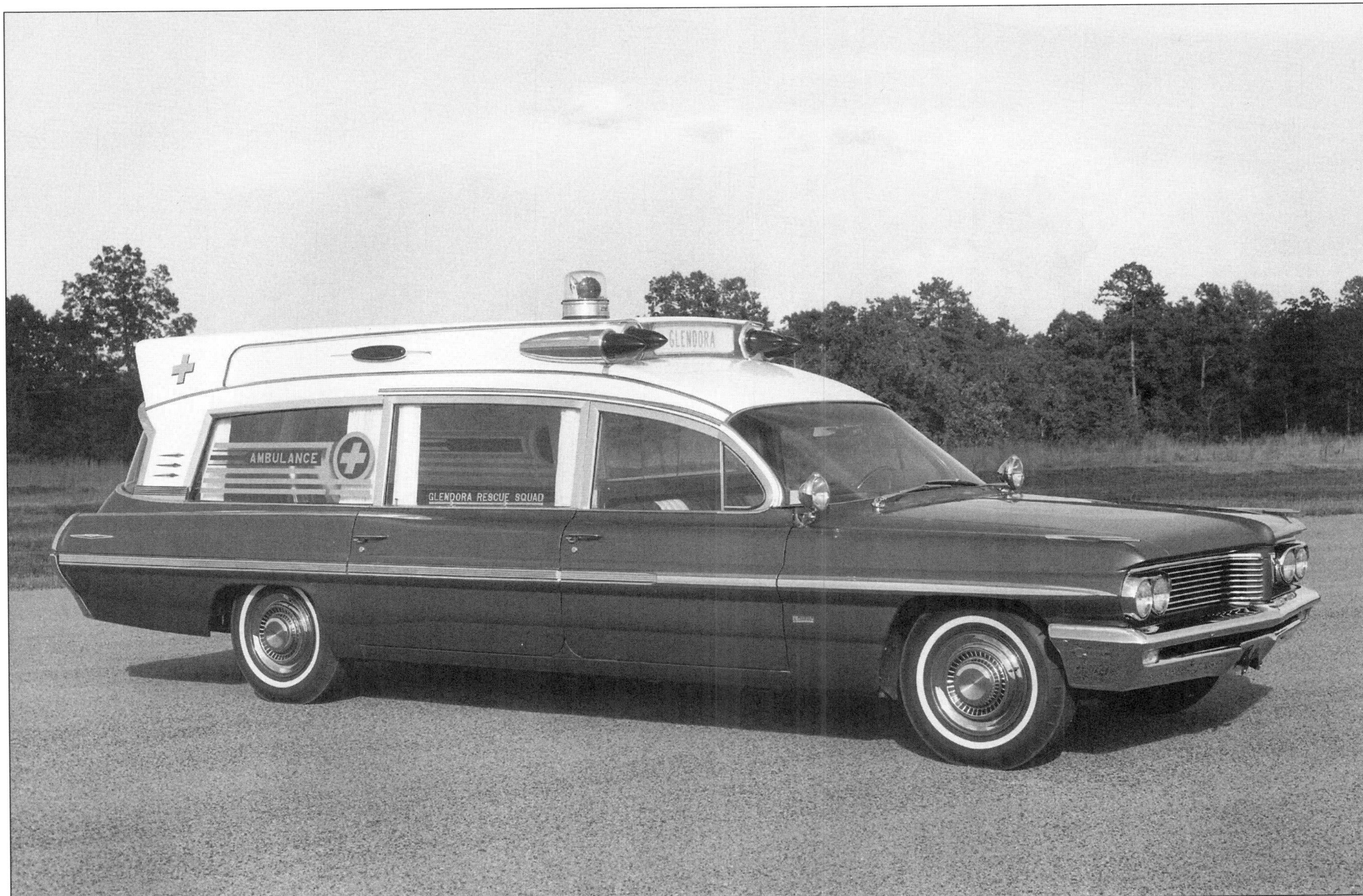

1962 SUPERIOR-PONTIAC CRITERION HIGHTOP AMBULANCE - Superior's Pontiac ambulances didn't take a rear seat to the company's significantly more expensive Cadillacs when it came to stunning good looks. This 1962 Superior-Pontiac Super Headroom 46-inch Ambulance was as good-looking as anything else on the road. This Superior-Pontiac Criterion was built for the Glendora (Pennsylvania) Rescue Squad.

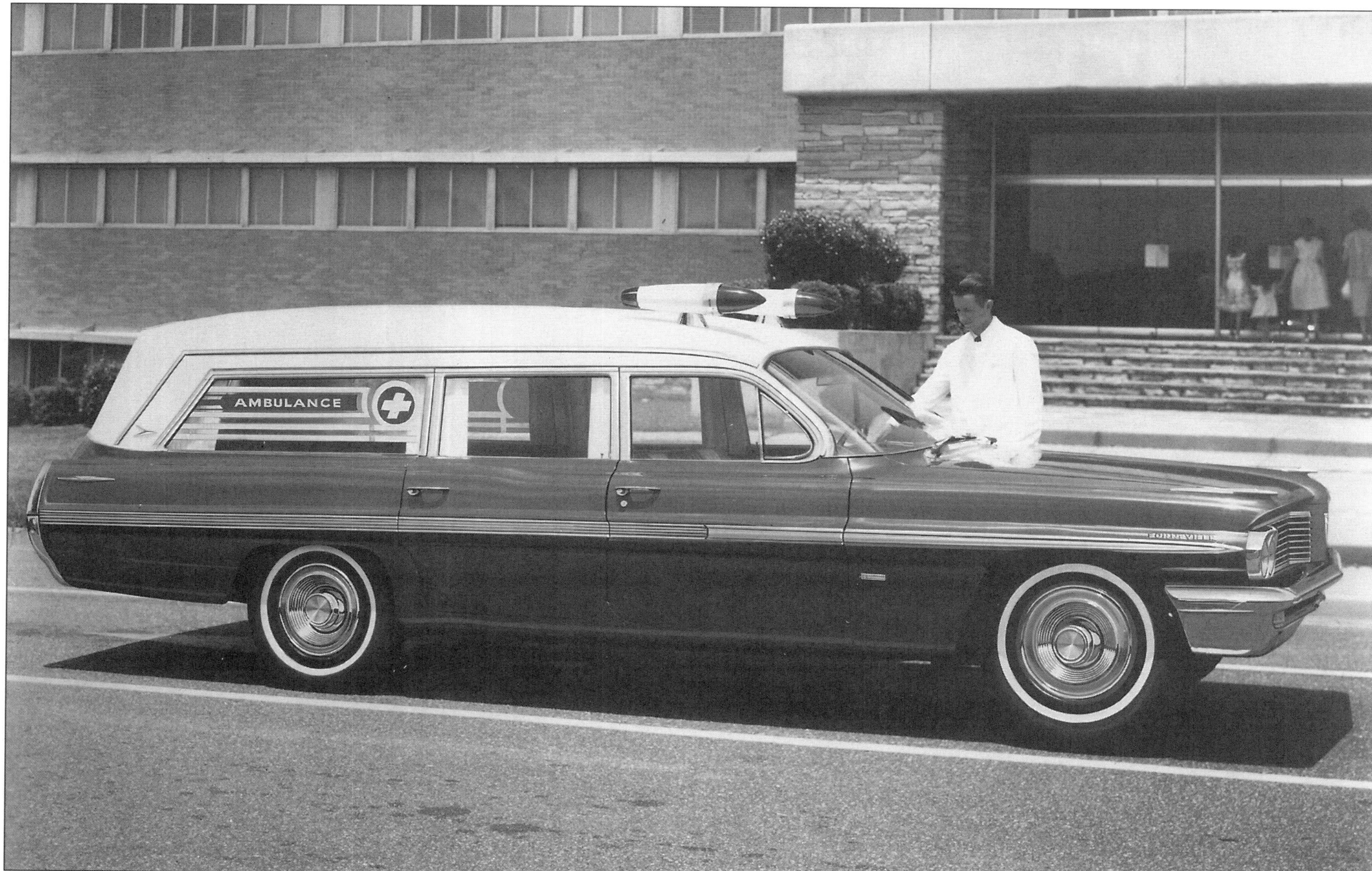

1962 SUPERIOR-PONTIAC CONSORT AMBULANCE - In mid-1961 the Superior Coach Corporation announced its all-new Consort series. Built on a standard wheelbase Pontiac Bonneville chassis with raised roof, the compact Consort was available in ambulance, funeral coach, combination and funeral service car models. With its white-over-red paint job and bullet-type roof lights, the Consort ambulance was a slick looking vehicle with performance to match.

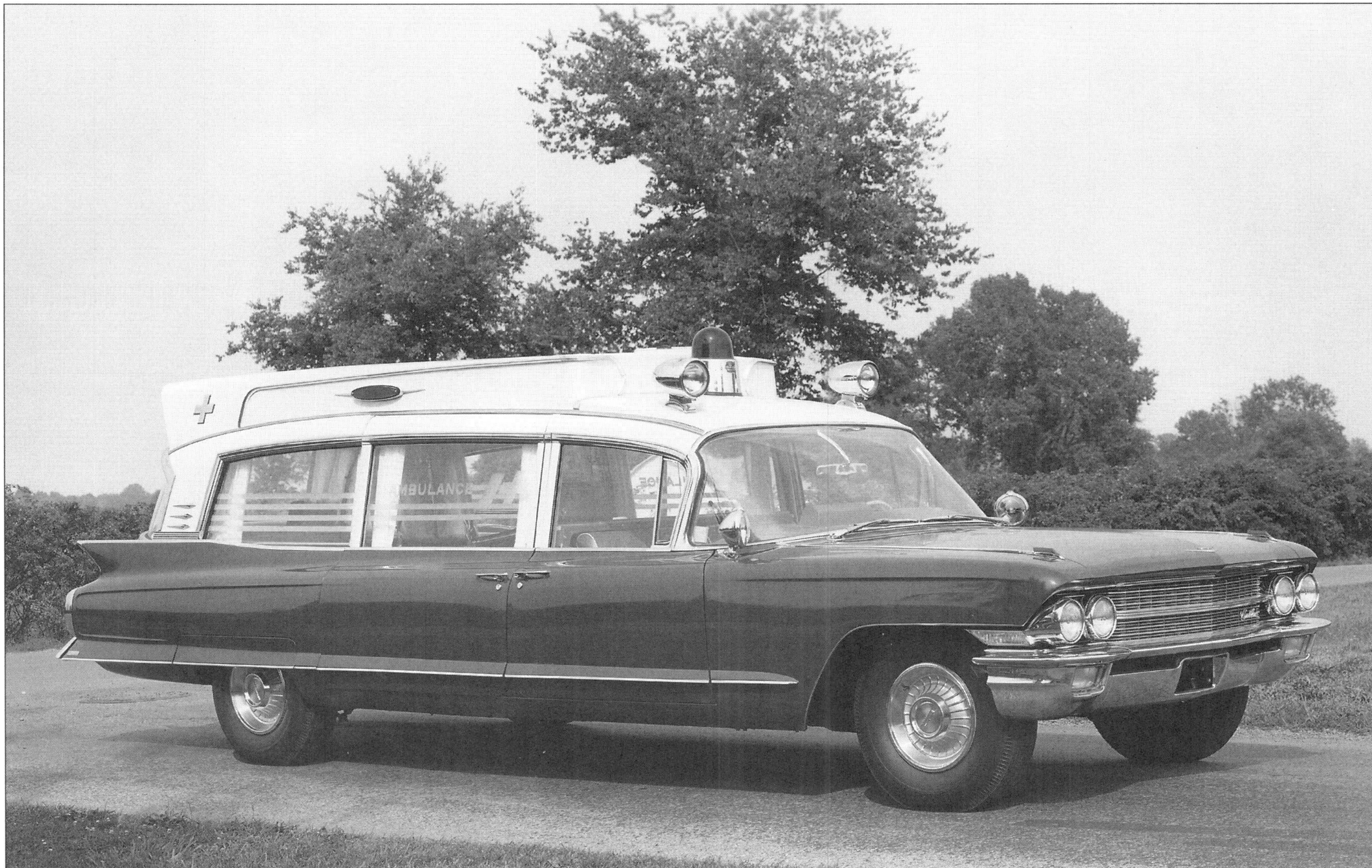

1962 SUPERIOR-CADILLAC ROYALE RESCUER - Positioned between the standard headroom Royale and the 54-inch Super Rescuer was Superior's 51-inch Rescuer Hightop ambulance. This 1962 Royale Rescuer wears black sidewall tires. Its roof is outfitted with two Federal Solar Ray white-lensed warning lights and a Beacon Ray mounted on an extra-high base to clear the raised roof.

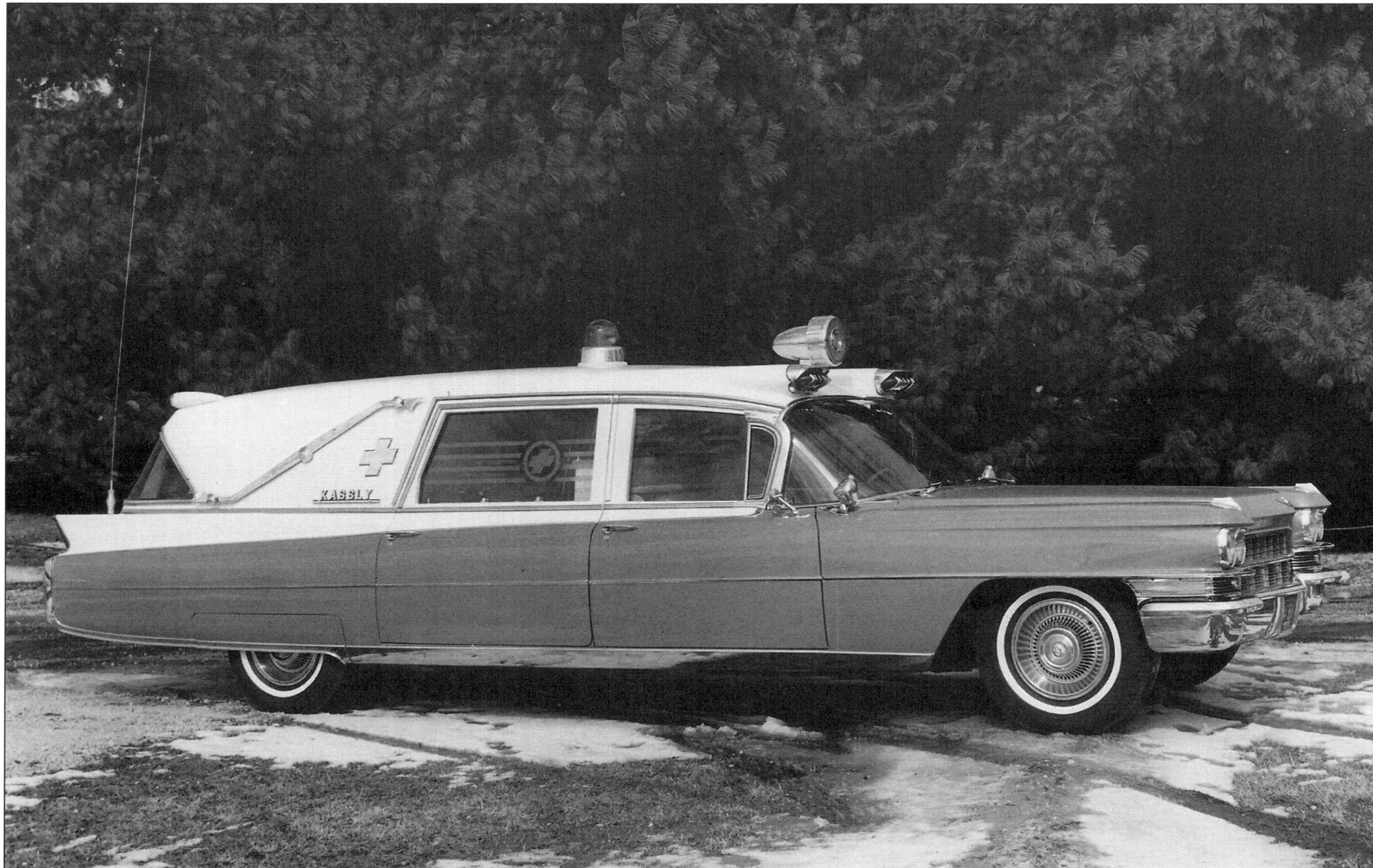

1963 EUREKA-CADILLAC LANDAU AMBULANCE - The most elegant offering in Eureka's 1963 Cadillac ambulance lineup was the Landau Ambulance. Utilizing the same body shell as the company's formal landau hearses, the Landau Ambulance featured closed rear quarter panels ornamented with large chrome landau bows. A plated cross emblem and "Kassly" nameplates are also mounted on the quarter panel. Note the triangular rear windows, quad flashers faired into the roof and the roof-mounted Federal "Q" siren.

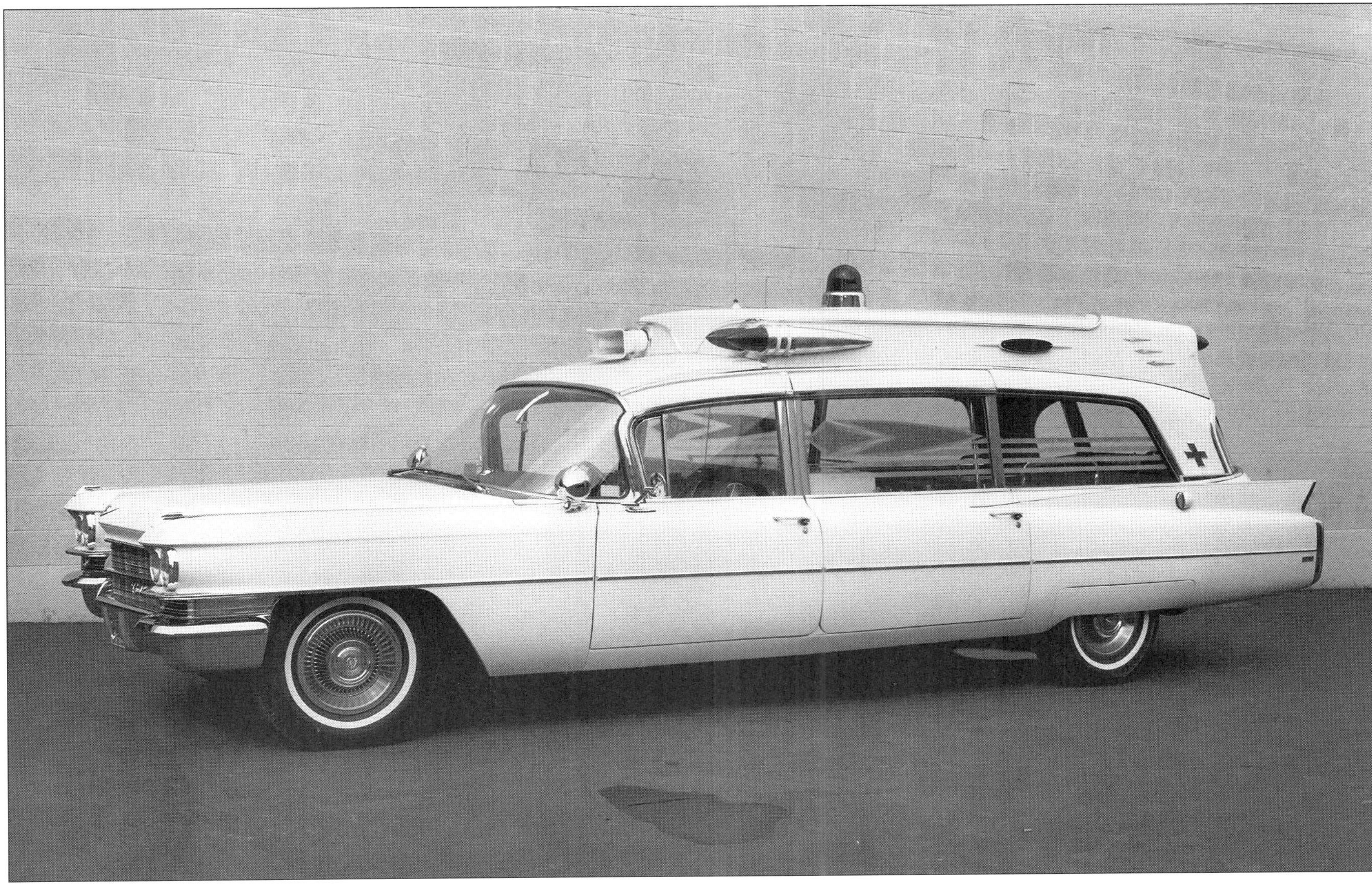

1963 SUPERIOR-CADILLAC ROYALE RESCUER - Superior's professional cars were extensively restyled in this year. This 1963 Royale Rescuer 50-inch Hightop Ambulance is equipped with Superior's trademark "bullet" red warning lights front and rear. An electronic siren/speaker is mounted above the windshield and a red-domed Federal Beacon Ray in the center of the raised fiberglass roof. The air scoop on the rear fender indicated that this ambulance is air-conditioned.

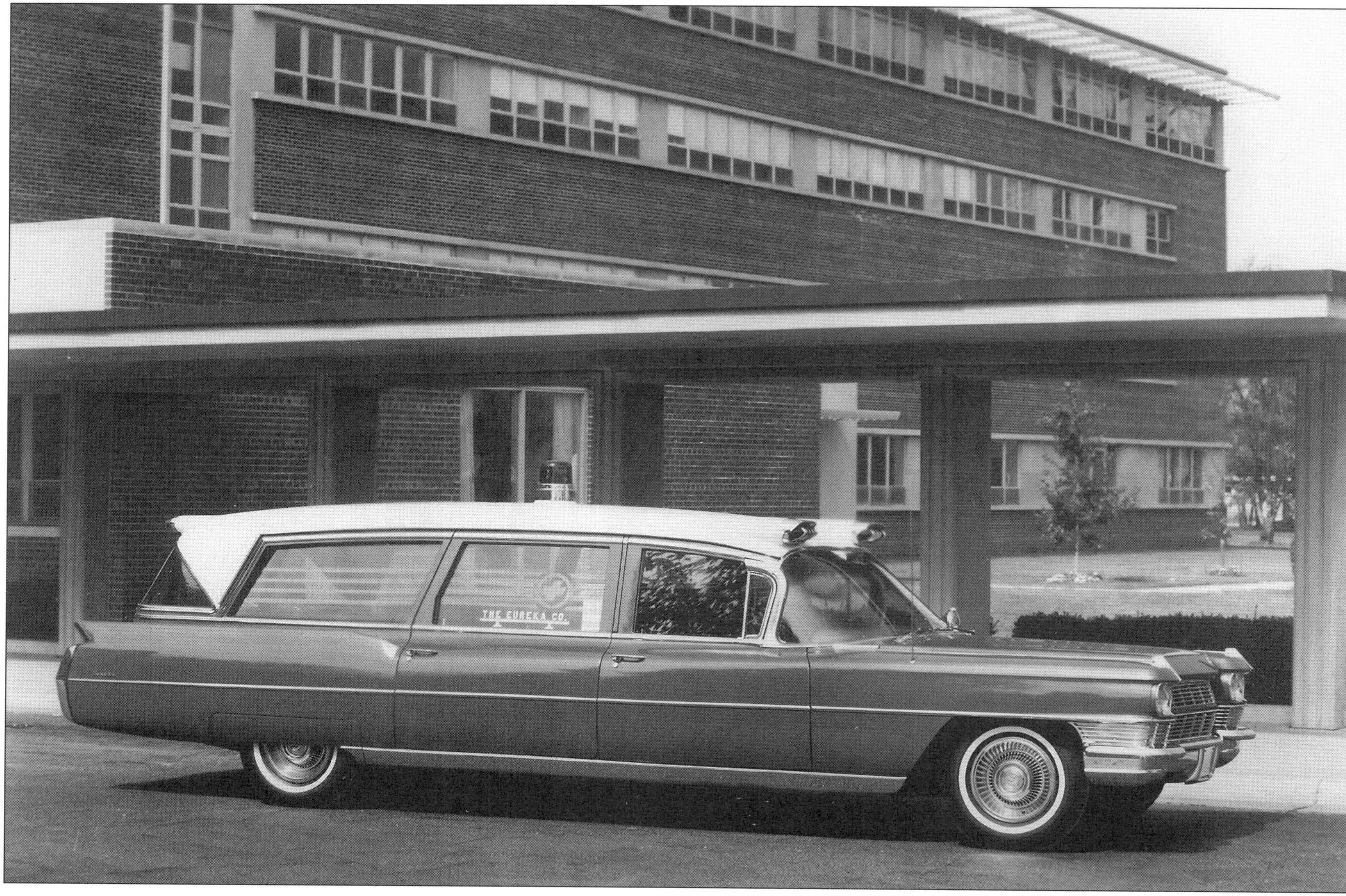

1964 EUREKA-CADILLAC AMBULANCE - The 1964 model year would be the last for The Eureka Company of Rock Falls, Illinois. Eureka's roots extended all the way back to 1887. Originally a manufacturer of furniture and buggies, Eureka had been building funeral cars and ambulances since 1917. This was The Eureka Company's standard limousine ambulance - the last of a long, proud line.

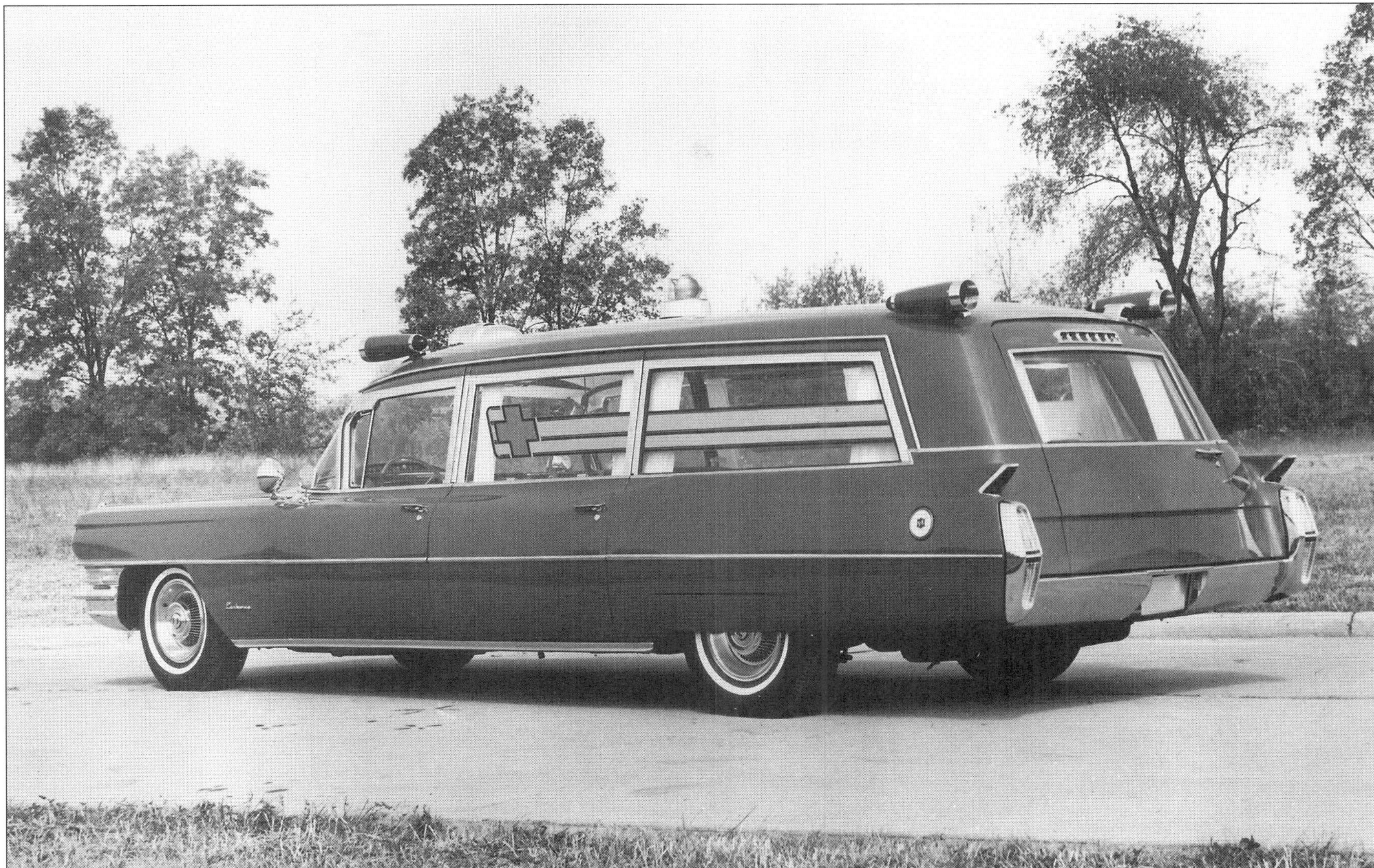

1964 S&S CADILLAC SUPERLINE PARKWAY AMBULANCE - The Hess & Eisenhardt Co. of Cincinnati was known for its premium S&S Cadillac funeral cars and ambulances. This is the standard-headroom (42.5-inch) S&S Superline Parkway Limousine Ambulance. Note the distinctive S&S Fyrball flashing red lights mounted on each corner of this car's roof, the prominent window striping and the Sayers & Scovill emblem incorporated into the fuel tank access door in the rear fender.

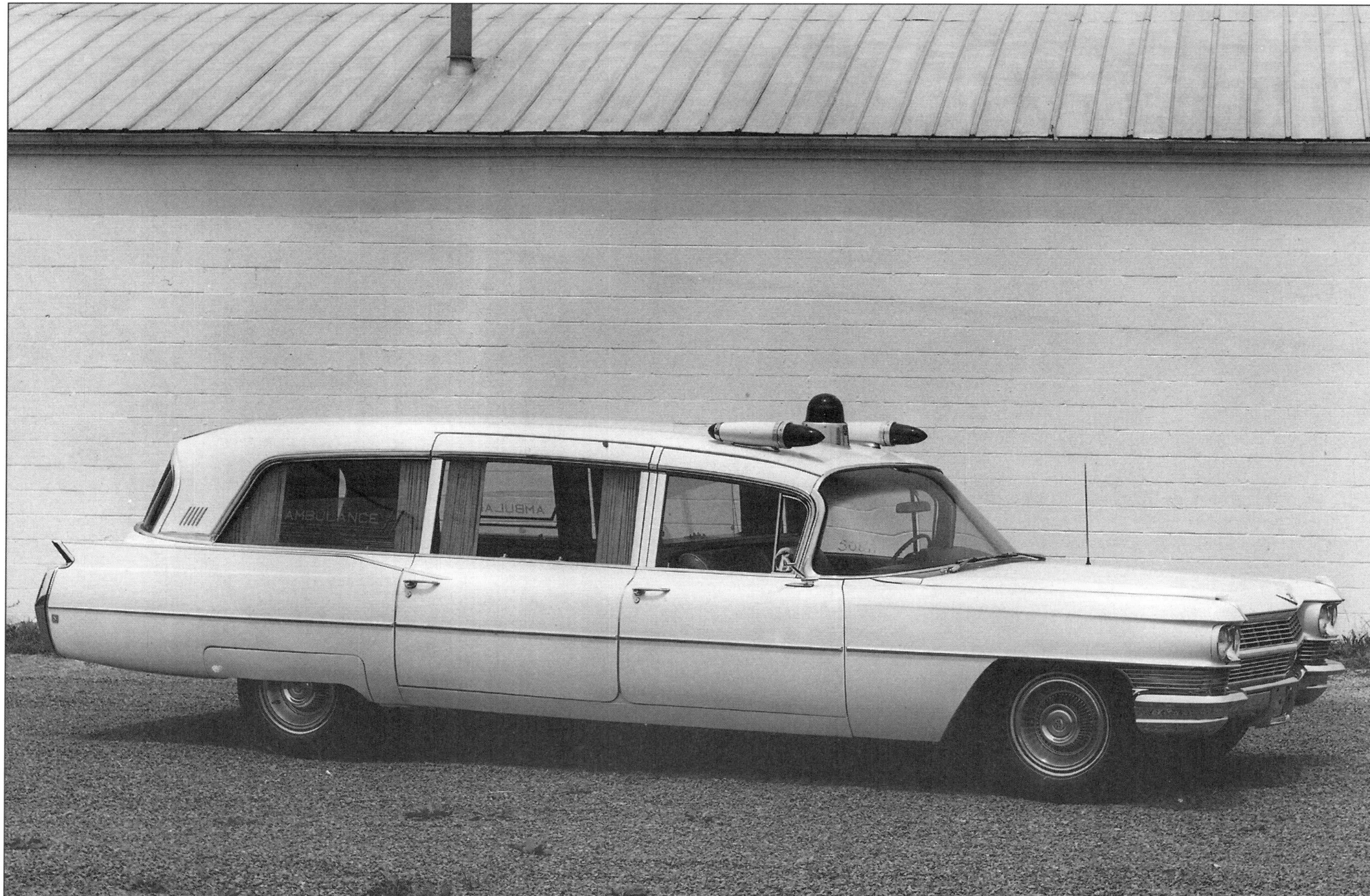

1964 SUPERIOR-CADILLAC ROYALE COMBINATION - The dual-purpose combination funeral coach/ambulance was the bread-and-butter of the American professional car industry. This versatile car could be converted from a hearse to an ambulance in minutes by adding the demountable roof lights and inserting Plexiglas "Ambulance" nameplates in the rear side windows. A quick-acting cot lock was mounted on the left wheelhouse cover.

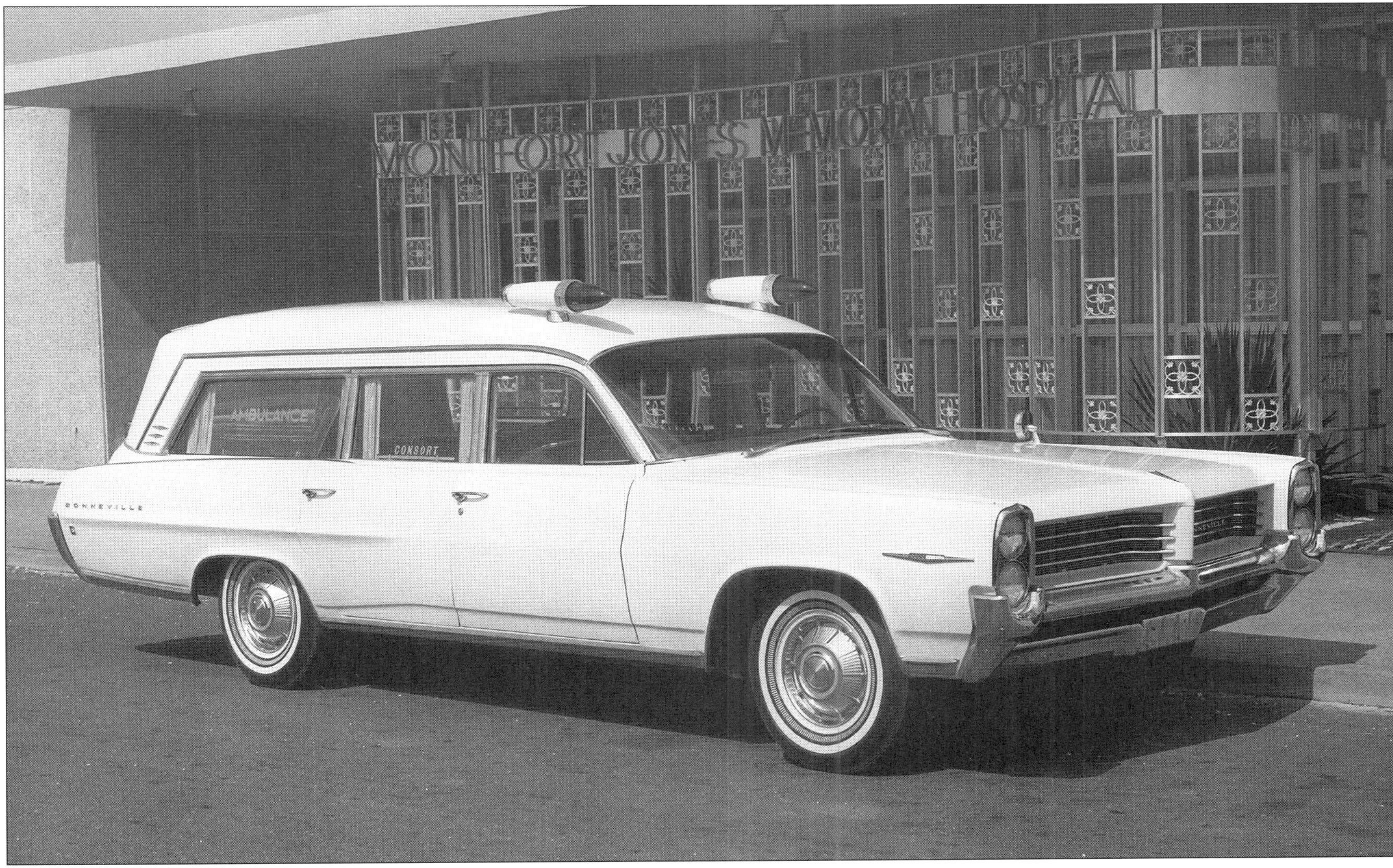

1964 SUPERIOR-PONTIAC CONSORT COMBINATION - Superior's compact Consort was well received by America's funeral directors, many of whom still provided local ambulance service. Built on a standard wheelbase Pontiac Bonneville chassis, the Consort was available in straight ambulance, funeral coach or combination funeral car/ambulance configurations. This is the basic Consort Limousine Combination in ambulance guise. The roof warning lights and "Ambulance" window signs could be quickly removed to convert this versatile vehicle into a funeral car.

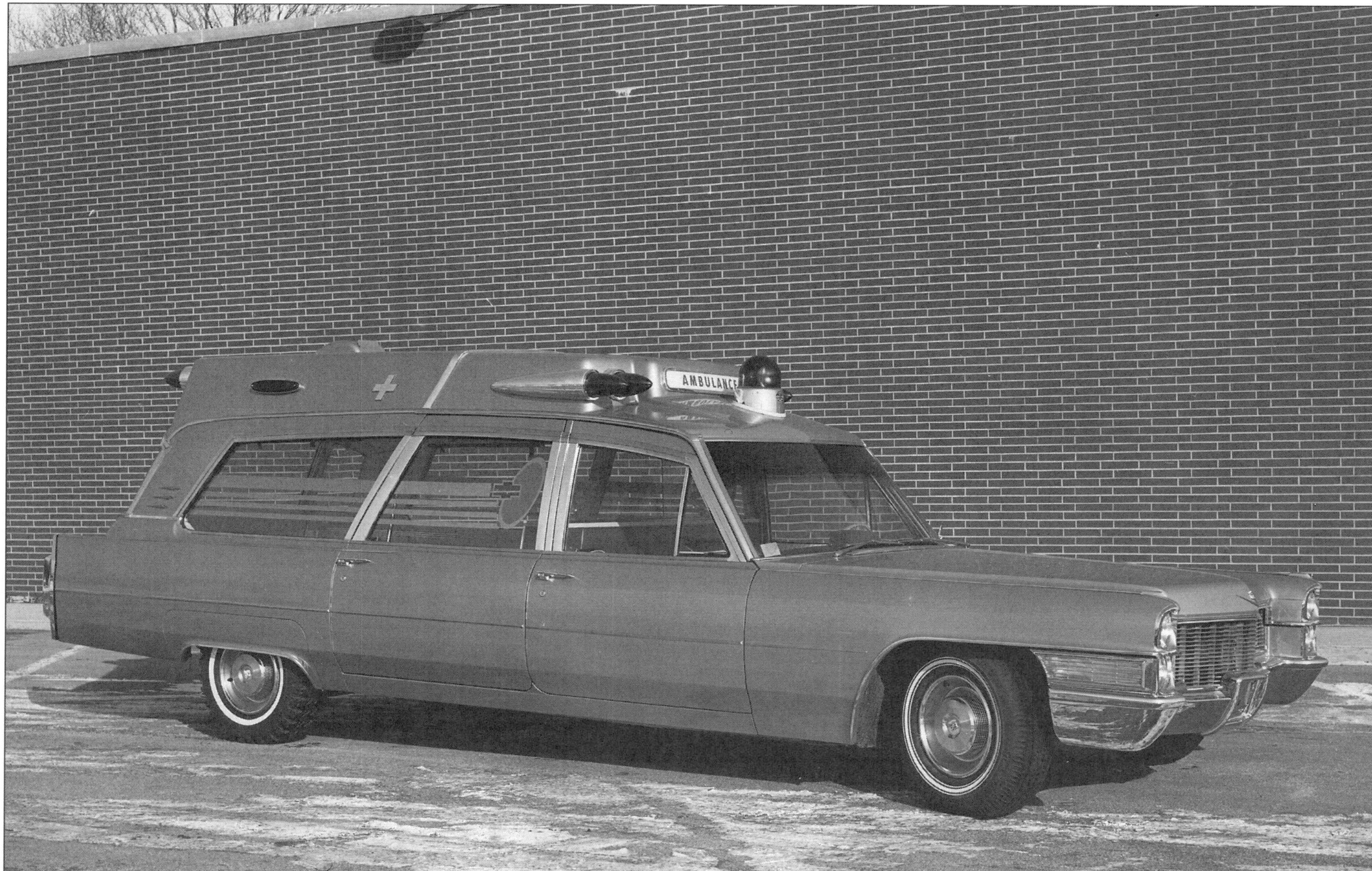

1965 SUPERIOR-CADILLAC RESCUER AMBULANCE - Cadillac completely redesigned its long-wheelbase commercial chassis for 1965. In addition to a new perimeter-type frame, the commercial chassis sported Cadillac's all-new exterior styling, which featured stacked headlights and finless rear fenders. This is the 1965 Superior Rescuer, which offered 51 inches of rear compartment headroom. Note the dual bullet-type flashing lights and roof ventilator.

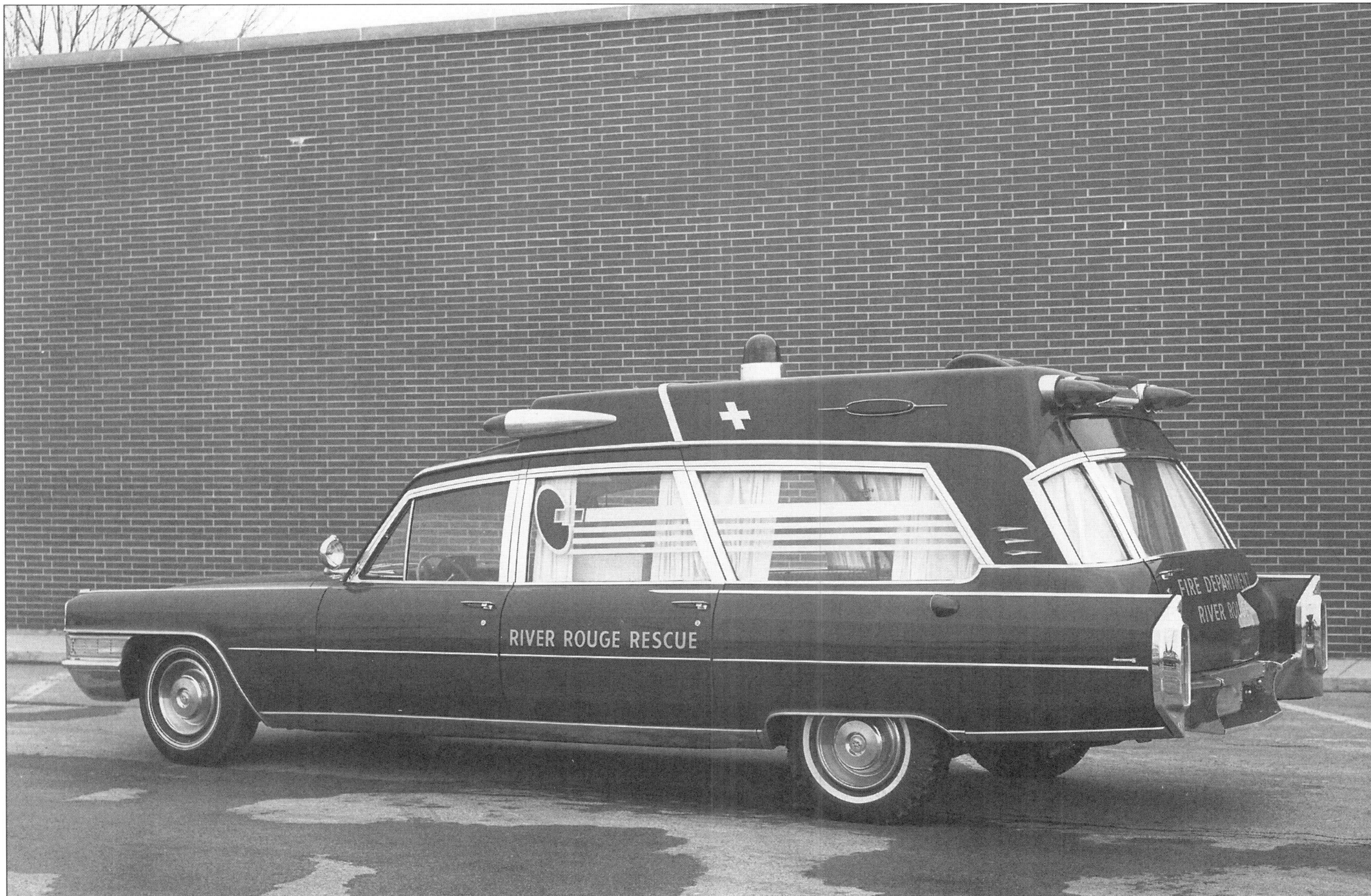

1965 SUPERIOR-CADILLAC RESCUER - This is a rear view of the 1965 Superior-Cadillac Rescuer 51-inch Ambulance delivered to the River Rouge, Michigan Fire Department Rescue Squad. This impressive high-headroom ambulance was painted a striking black-over-red. The angled “C” and “D” pillars and window striping give this emergency vehicle an illusion of speed even when it’s standing still!

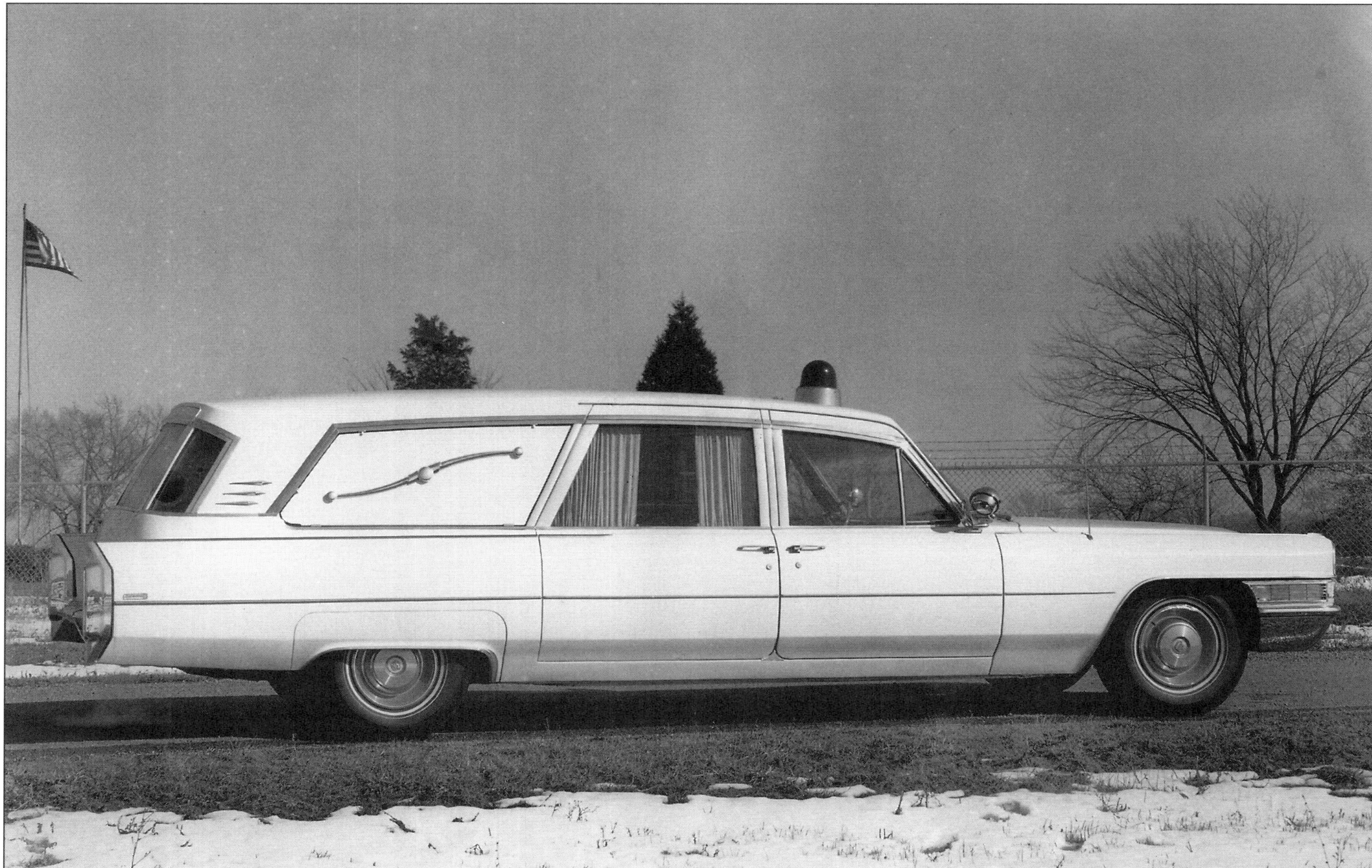

1965 SUPERIOR-CADILLAC ROYALE LIMOUSINE COMBINATION - Here's another Combination Coach. This 1965 Superior-Cadillac Royale Combination is outfitted as a Landau Funeral Coach. Removal of the landau panels in the rear side windows instantly converted this dual-purpose car into a smart Limousine Ambulance. Most combination coaches were painted neutral colors such as white, silver-grey or light metallic blue. Note the rear-hinged side doors and the small rear quarter windows.

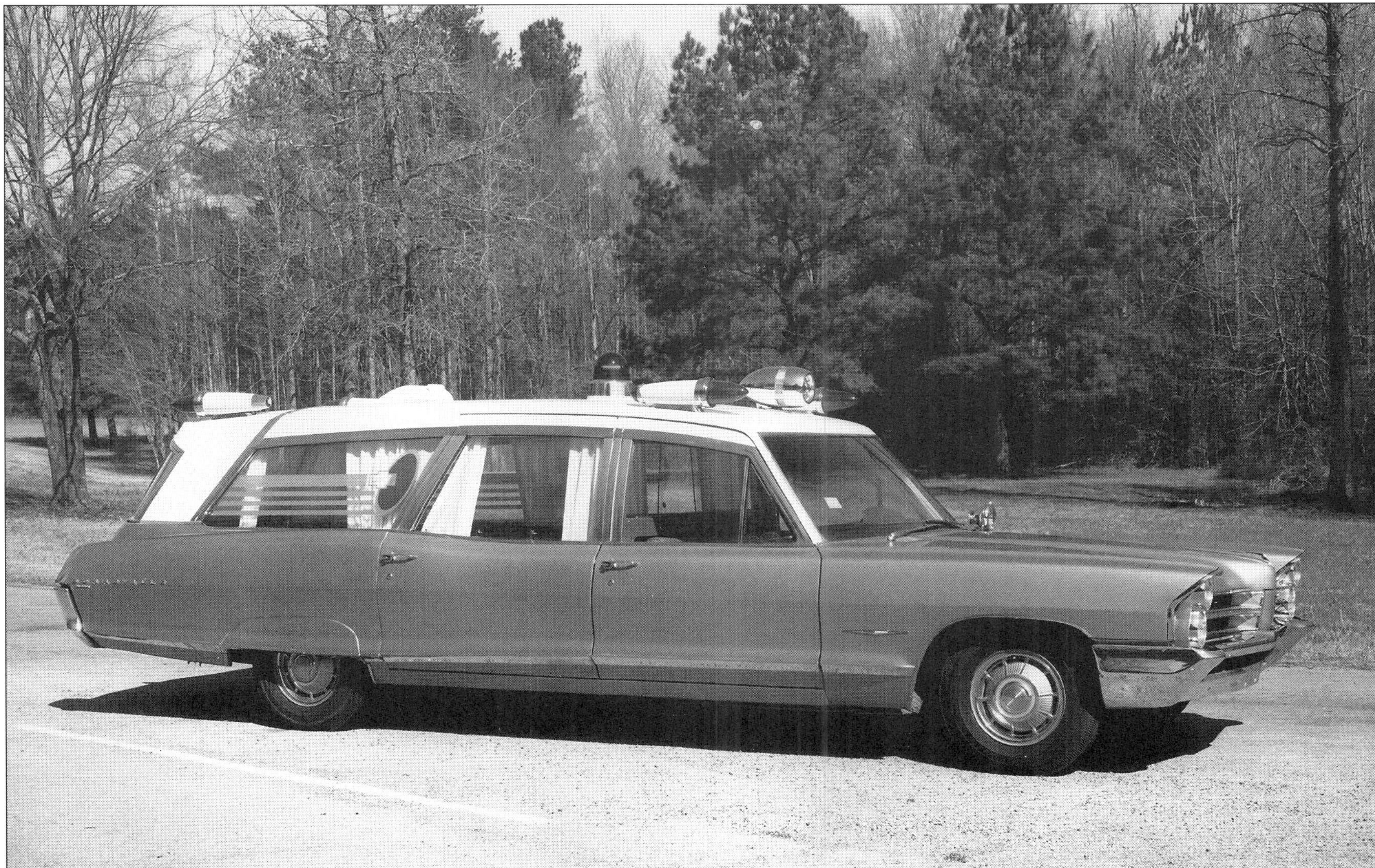

1965 SUPERIOR-PONTIAC AMBULANCE - Is it just us, or were these Pontiac chassied ambulances getting better looking every year? There's no question that Superior's less-expensive Pontiacs were every bit as attractively styled as their big-brother Cadillacs. This 1965 Superior Pontiac 40-inch Ambulance is a case in point. With the increasing popularity of electronic sirens and speakers, the roof-mounted coaster siren was becoming something of a rarity.

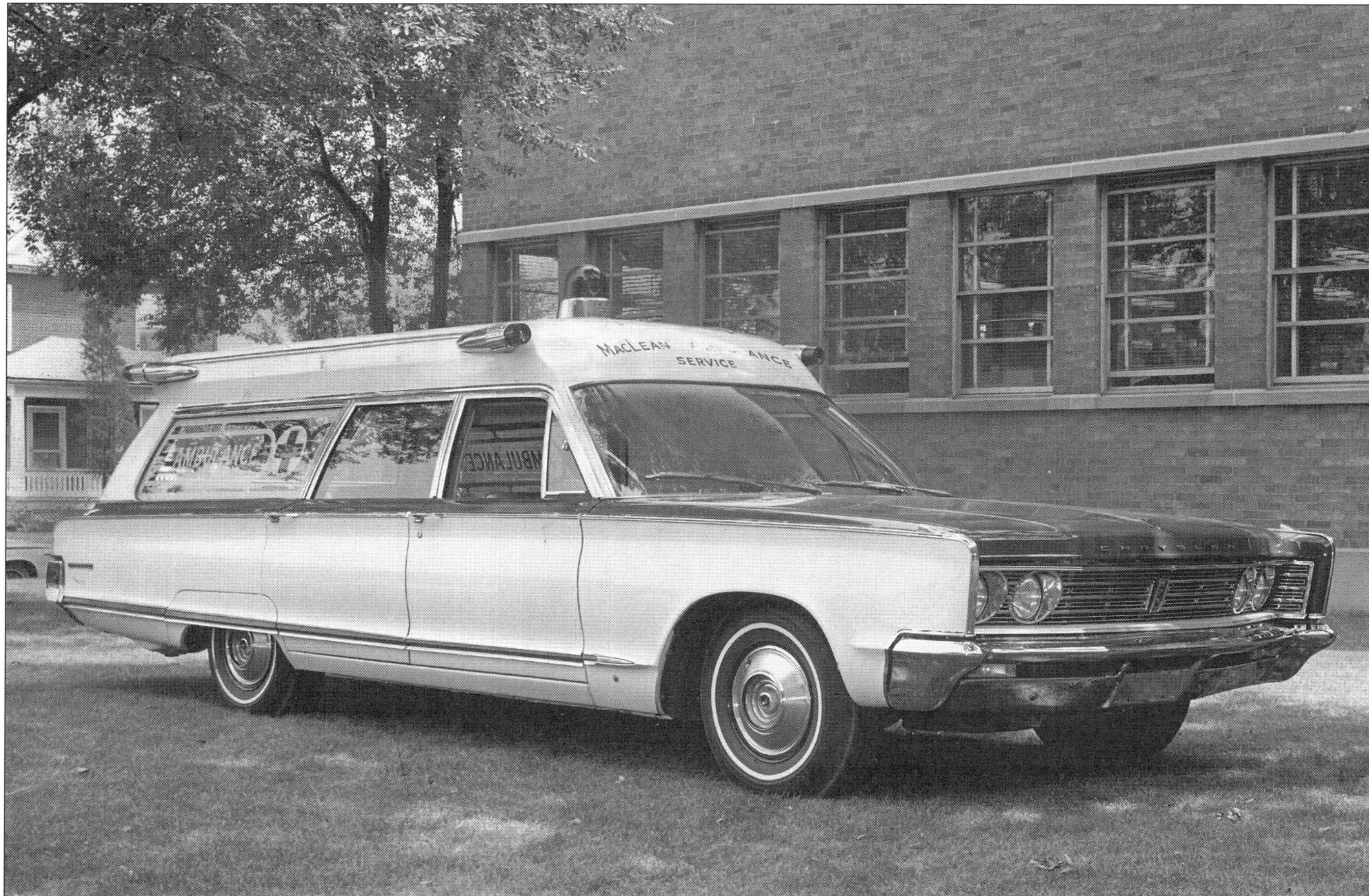

1965 RENAUD-CHRYSLER AMBULANCE - A small local builder, Paul Renaud of Windsor, Ontario, Canada, built this handsome one-off ambulance. The base car was a 1965 Chrysler Newport Station Wagon. Renaud literally "raised the roof" to create a high-headroom ambulance for the MacLean Ambulance Service in Canada's Maritime Provinces.

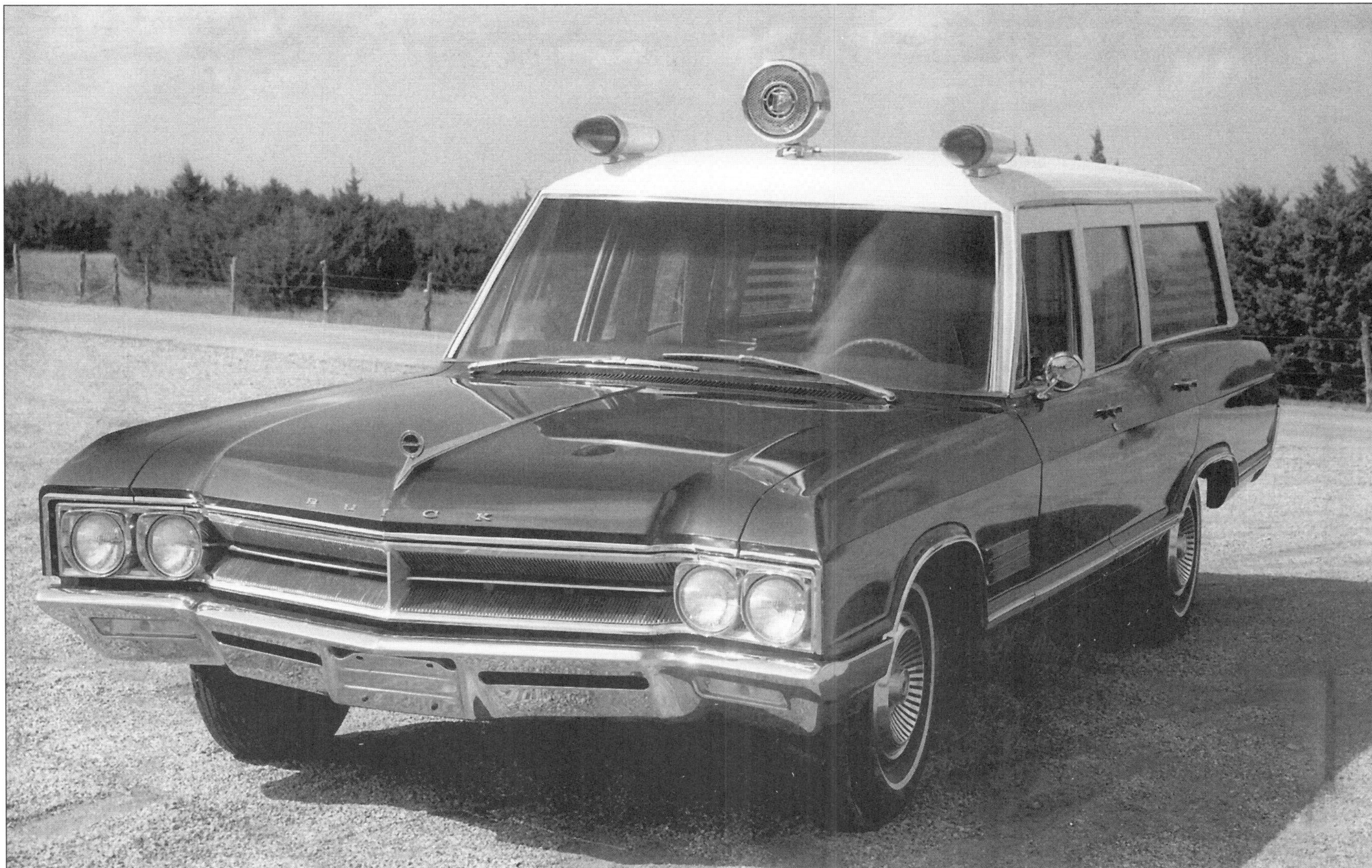

1965 TRINITY-BUICK AMBULANCE - The Flxible Company of Loudonville, Ohio, ceased funeral car and ambulance production for the second and final time early in the 1965 model year. A new company, Trinity Coach of Duncanville, Texas, took over Buick professional car production where Flxible left off. This is a Trinity-Buick Ambulance on the 1965 Buick Wildcat chassis. Note the commercial windshield glass (flat instead of curved), side window glass and the Federal "Q" siren mounted on the roof. Within four years, Trinity was gone, too.

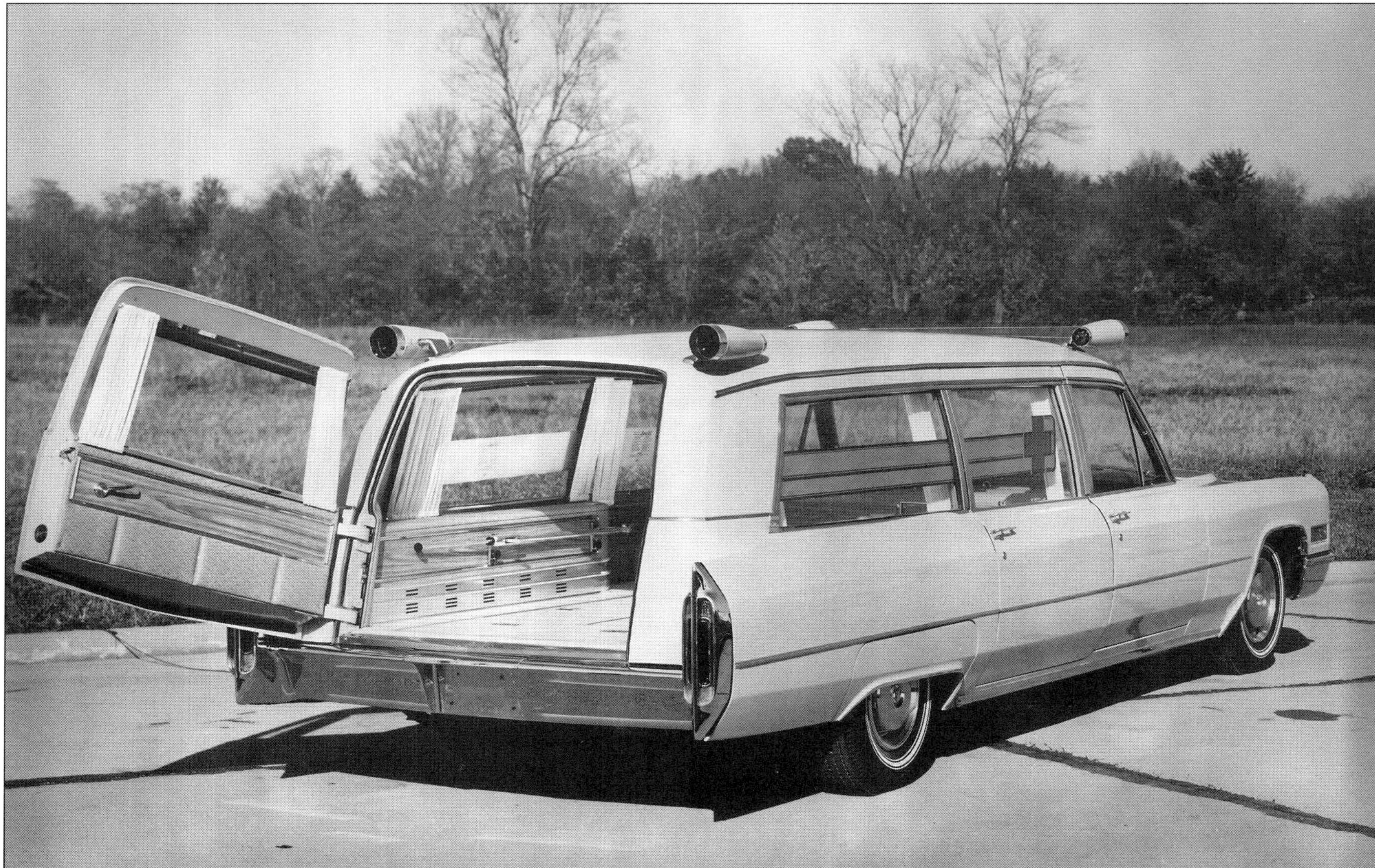

1966 S&S CADILLAC PARKWAY AMBULANCE - The Hess & Eisenhardt Company again offered three S&S Cadillac ambulance models: the standard-headroom S&S Parkway, the raised-roof Kensington 48-inch and the high-headroom Custom Professional. This is a view of the business end of a 1966 S&S Cadillac Parkway Ambulance. The cot lock is visible on the left side wheelhouse. S&S professional cars were equipped with standard airline-type window drapes.

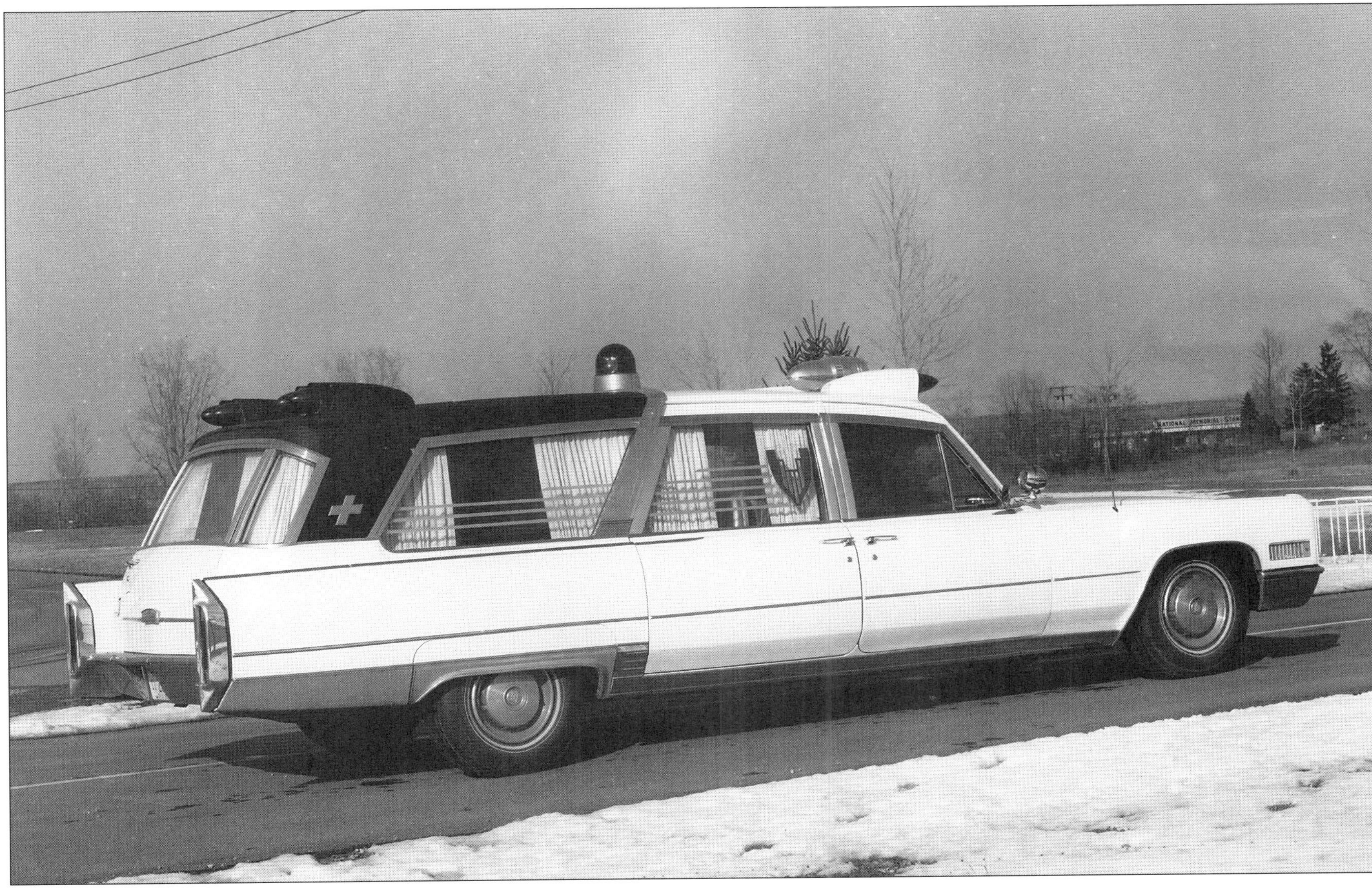

1966 SUPERIOR-CADILLAC CROWN ROYALE LIMOUSINE AMBULANCE - The Superior Coach Corporation of Lima, Ohio, continued to offer a wide array of ambulance models on Pontiac and Cadillac chassis. Superior's premium series was the prestigious Crown Royale with its distinctive up-and-over "C"-pillar roof molding. This is the standard headroom (42-inch) 1966 Superior-Cadillac Crown Royale Limousine Ambulance. The rear roof area has a black crinkle finish.

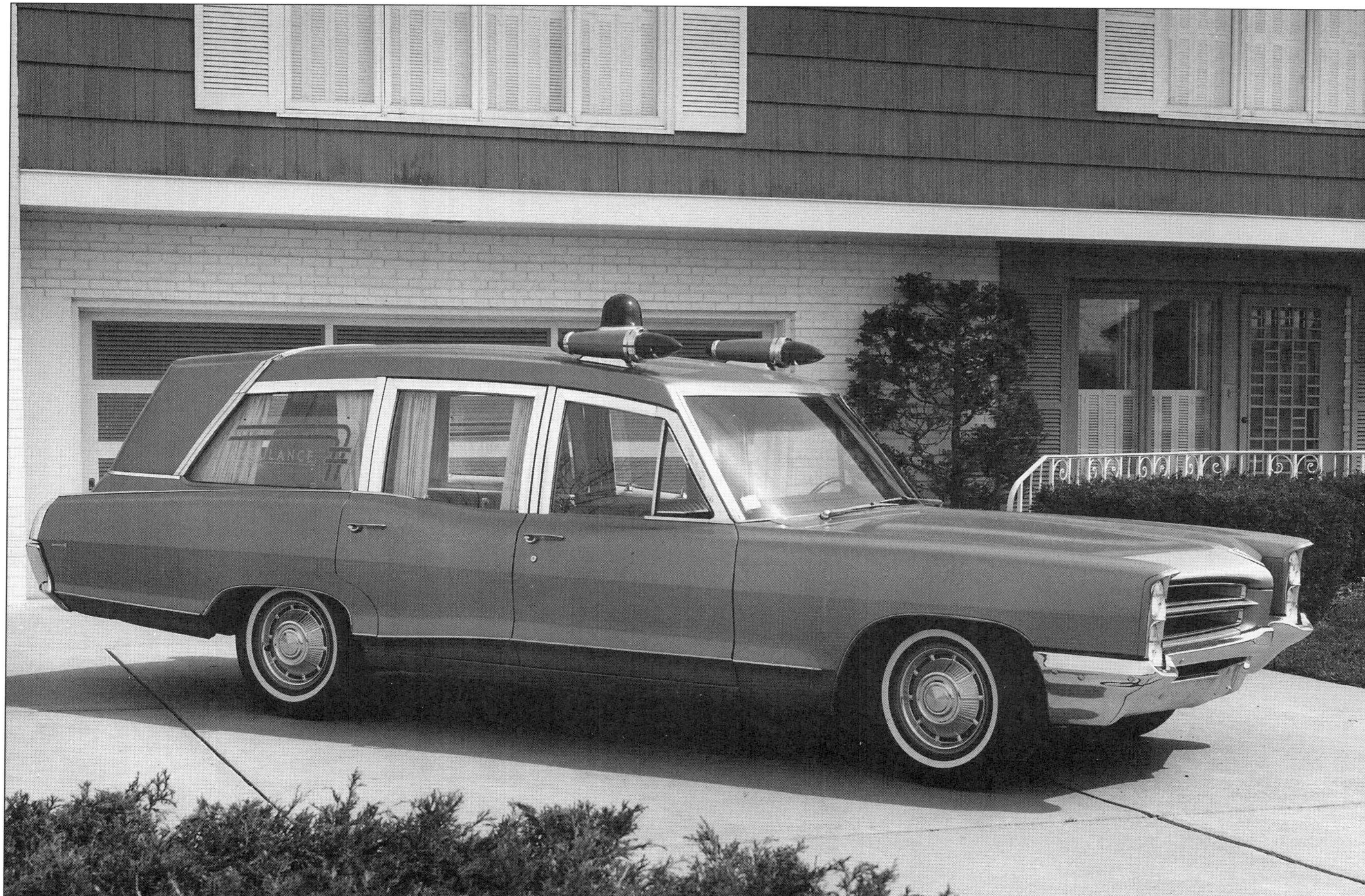

1966 SUPERIOR-PONTIAC CONSORT COMBINATION- Superior's 1966 Pontiac ambulances sported a distinctive new "Tiara" rear roof treatment on both standard and long-wheelbase chassis. The translucent "Ambulance" panels in the rear side windows show that this 1966 Superior-Pontiac Consort was a combination coach that did double-duty as a funeral car or ambulance.

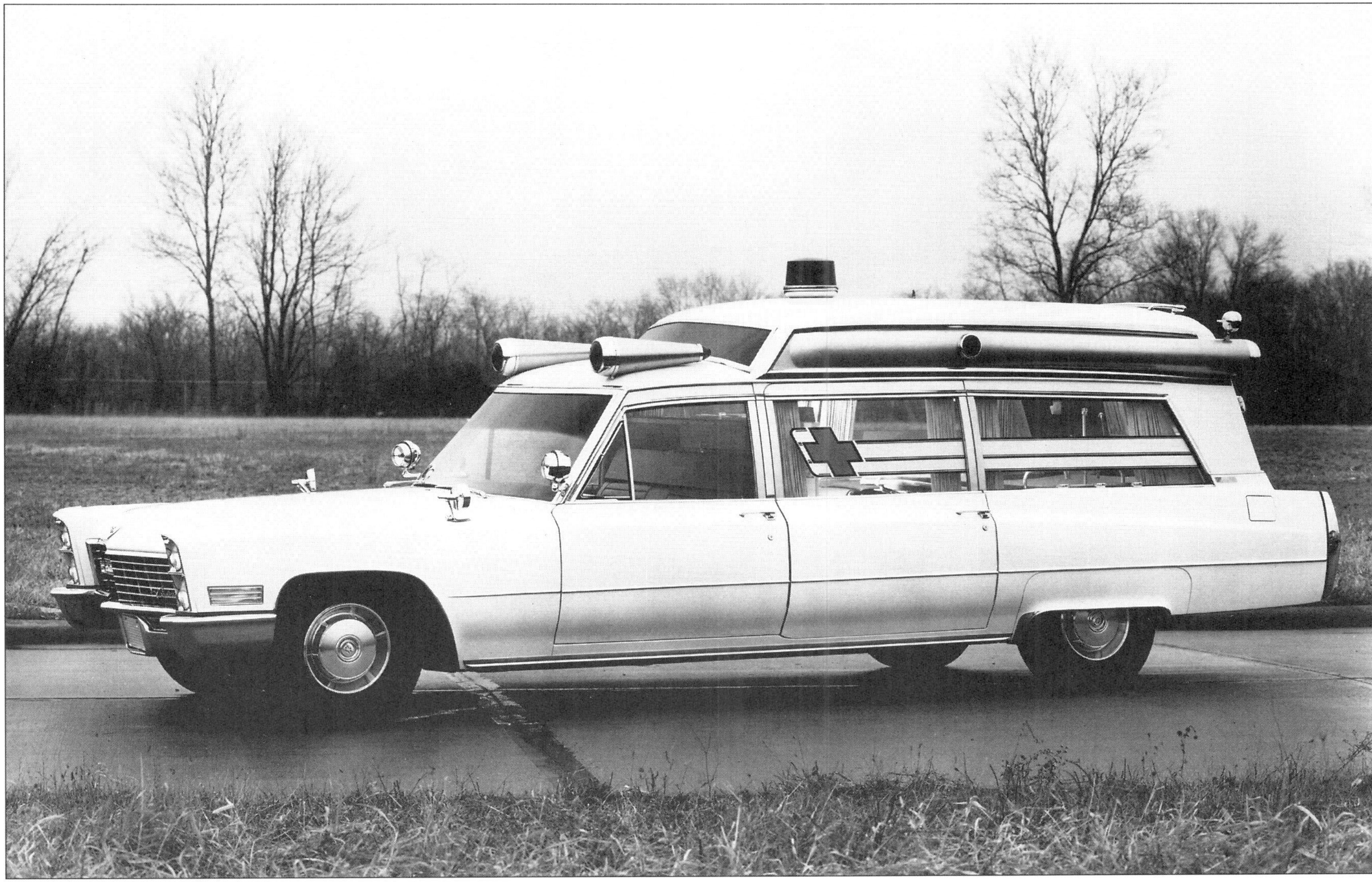

1967 S&S CADILLAC PROFESSIONAL HIGH-BODY AMBULANCE - The Hess & Eisenhardt Company's top-line ambulance was the imposing S&S Cadillac Professional High Body. With 54 inches of headroom in its rear compartment, the Professional High Body was instantly distinguishable from its lesser siblings by its tubular stainless steel upper body trim (which housed seven-inch red rear roof flashers) and the illuminated Plexiglas panel in the front of its step-type roof. The conical tunnel lights over the cab also hold seven-inch red flashing lights.

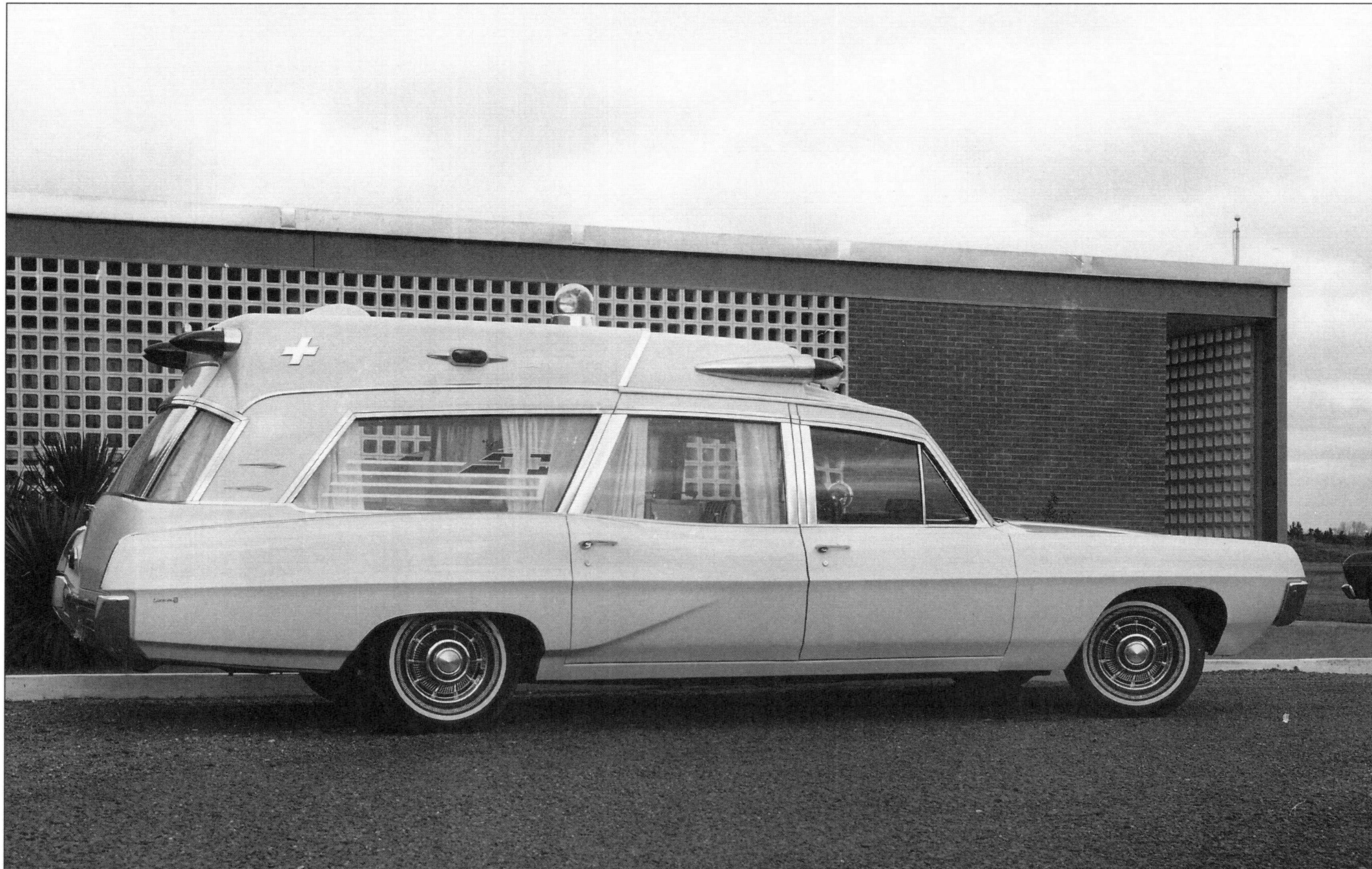

1967 SUPERIOR-PONTIAC HIGH-HEADROOM AMBULANCE - Superior built its passenger car-based ambulances in two separate production facilities. Superior-Cadillac ambulances were built in the company's home plant in Lima, Ohio. All of the company's Pontiac ambulances were built in the Southern Division plant in Kosiusko, Mississippi. This is a gleaming white 1967 Superior Pontiac 48-inch High-Headroom Ambulance. Note the distinctive Superior bullet lights front and rear, and the clear-domed Beacon Ray roof light.

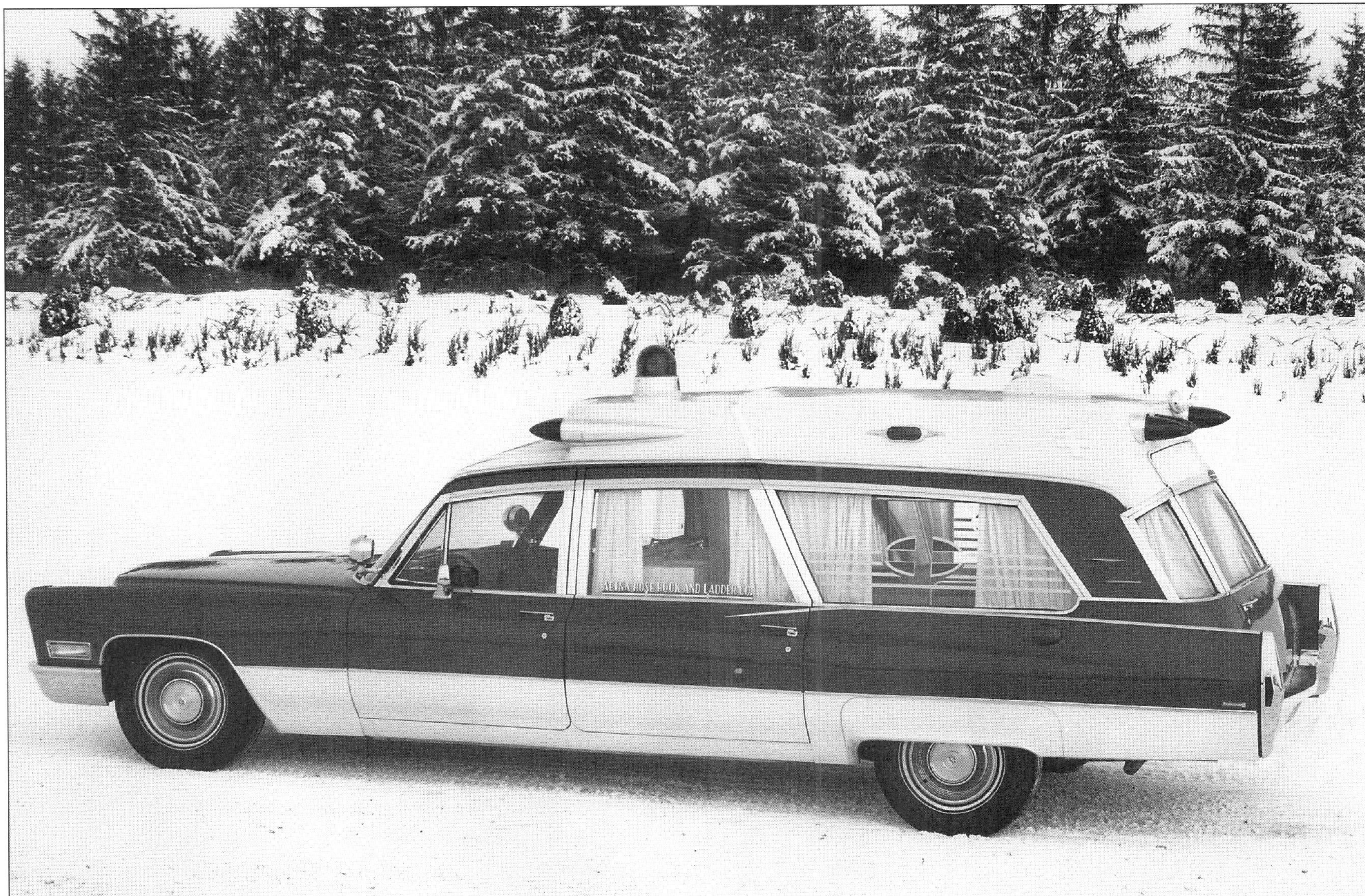

1968 SUPERIOR-CADILLAC RESCUER AMBULANCE - Superior continued to offer a choice of three Cadillac-chassised ambulances with different rear compartment headroom heights. This is the top-line 51-inch Superior-Cadillac Rescuer. Note the airline-style window drapes and two-tone paint job. This Rescuer was built for a fire company: the Aetna Hook & Ladder Company.

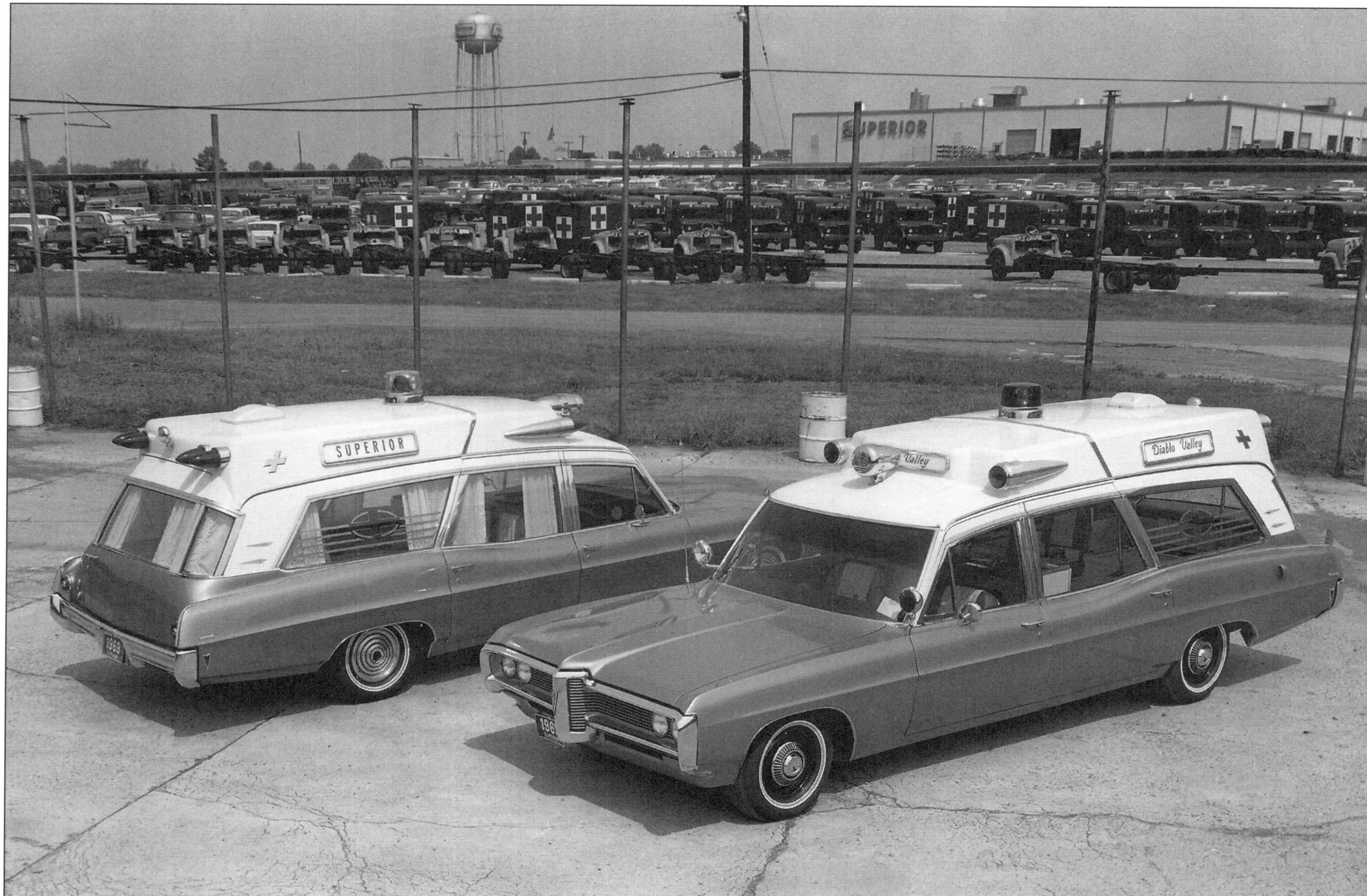

1968 SUPERIOR-PONTIAC HIGHTOP AMBULANCES - This interesting photograph, taken at Superior's Southern Division plant in Kosiusko, Mississippi, features both front and rear views of Superior's 1968 Pontiac High-Headroom Ambulance. Both of these ambulances are equipped with roof-mounted coaster sirens and Superior's bullet-shaped rear warning lights. The unit on the right was delivered to the Diablo Valley Ambulance Service.

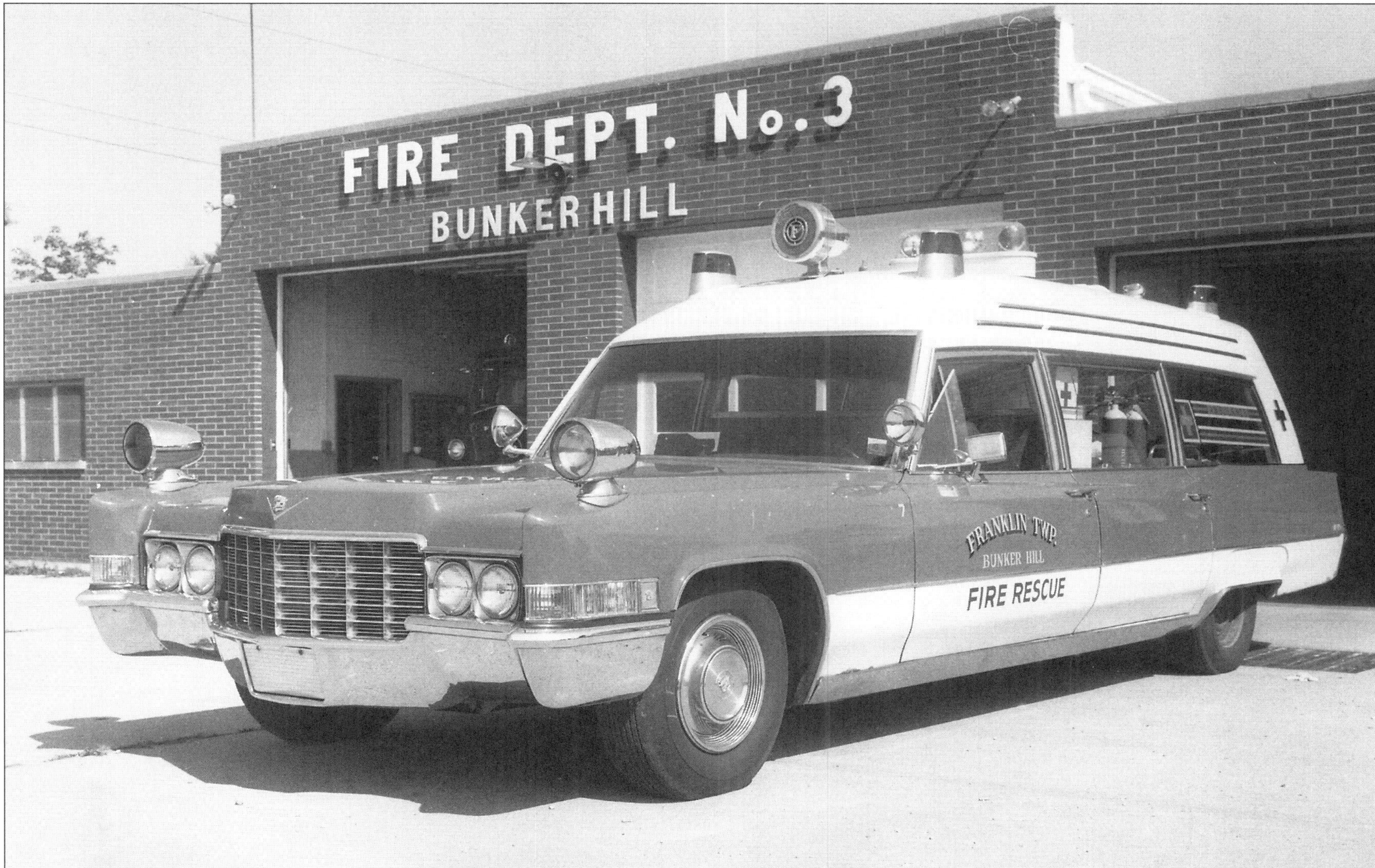

1969 MILLER-METEOR CADILLAC CLASSIC 48 AMBULANCE - The Miller-Meteor Division of the Divco-Wayne Corp. offered two Cadillac ambulances for 1969. Miller-Meteor's premium model was the 48-inch high headroom Classic 48 shown here. Operated by the Bunker Hill Fire Department of Franklin Township Indiana, this M/M Classic 48 is equipped with M/M's unique Ful-Vu 360-degree red flashing lights at each corner, an Aurora Borealis in the middle of the roof, and a Federal "Q" siren. Fender-mounted Propello-Rays also helped clear the way.

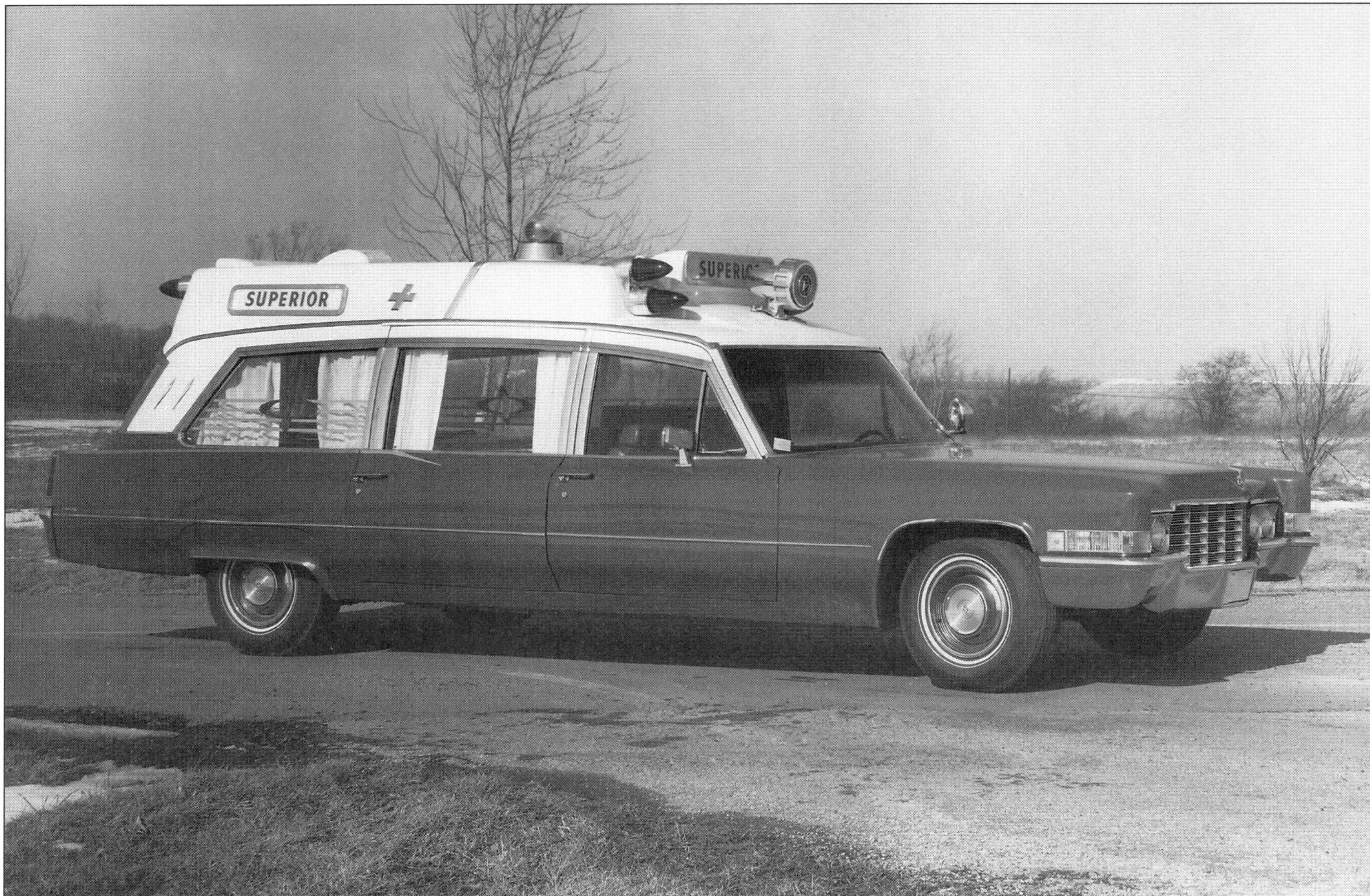

1969 SUPERIOR-CADILLAC RESCUER AMBULANCE - Despite the wide acceptance of electronic sirens, many emergency vehicle operators still preferred mechanical sirens like Federal's ubiquitous "Q". This 1969 Superior-Cadillac 51-inch Rescuer is equipped with a Q2B mounted in the center of the roof, canted quad bullet lights, and optional illuminated name panels on the front and sides of the fiberglass roof.

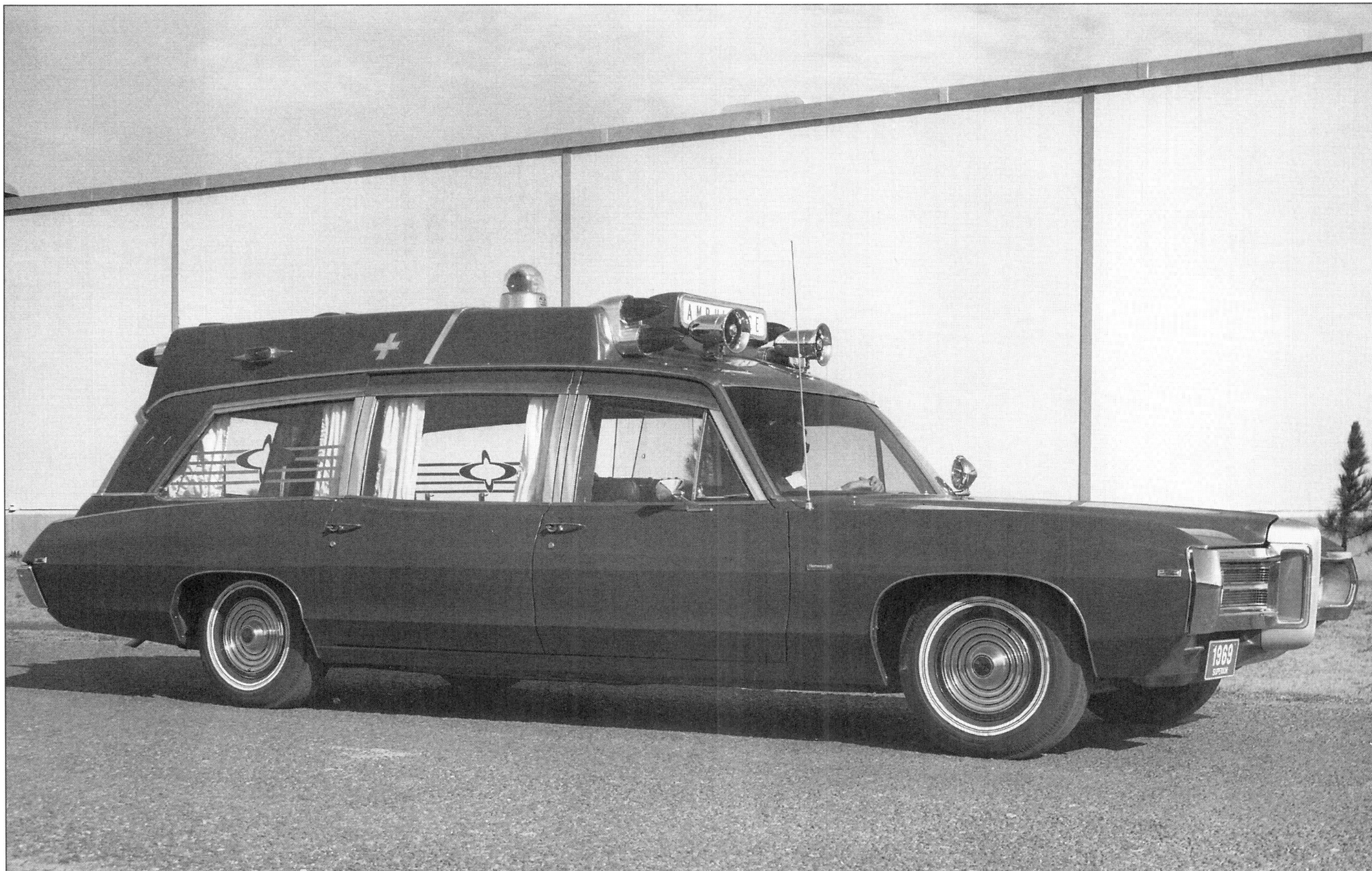

1969 SUPERIOR-PONTIAC HIGH-HEADROOM AMBULANCE - In addition to its premium Cadillacs, the Superior Coach Corp. (which was acquired by Sheller-Globe in this year) continued to offer a lower-priced series of ambulances on standard and extended-wheelbase Pontiac chassis. This is the top-line Pontiac, the 48-inch 1969 Superior-Pontiac High Headroom Ambulance. Superior's other Pontiac ambulances included a standard-headroom 40-incher and the compact, standard-wheelbase Consort.

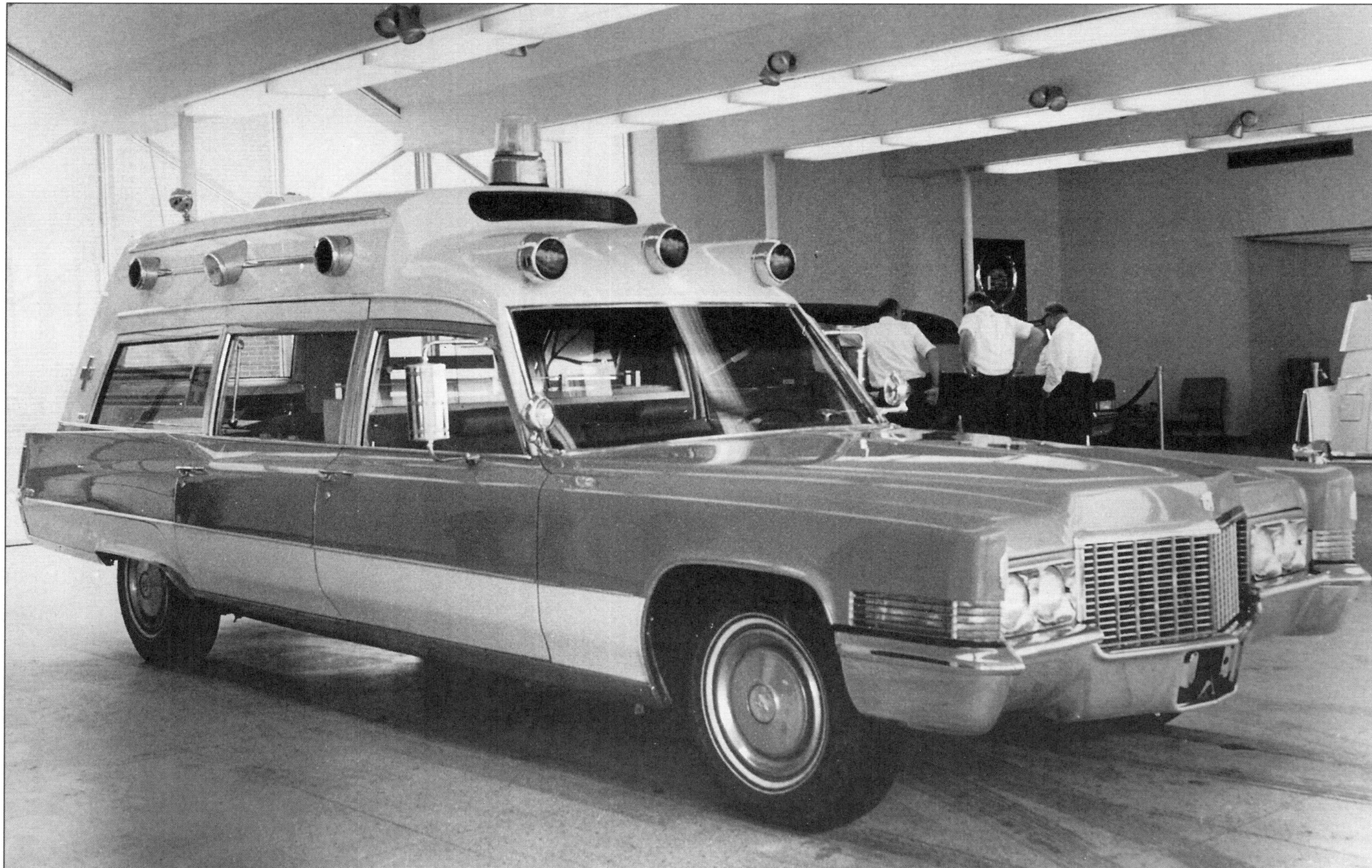

1970 MILLER-METEOR CADILLAC LIFELINER - Miller-Meteor offered no fewer than *four* Cadillac ambulances this year: the 42-inch Guardian, 48-inch Volunteer, 50-inch Interceptor and a new top-line professional Cadillac ambulance: the 54-inch Lifeliner shown here. This brand new M/M Lifeliner awaits delivery to its purchaser in the Miller-Meteor factory showroom in Piqua, Ohio. Note the triple tunnel lights, illuminated name panel, side mounted "ditch" lights and the West Coast mirrors.

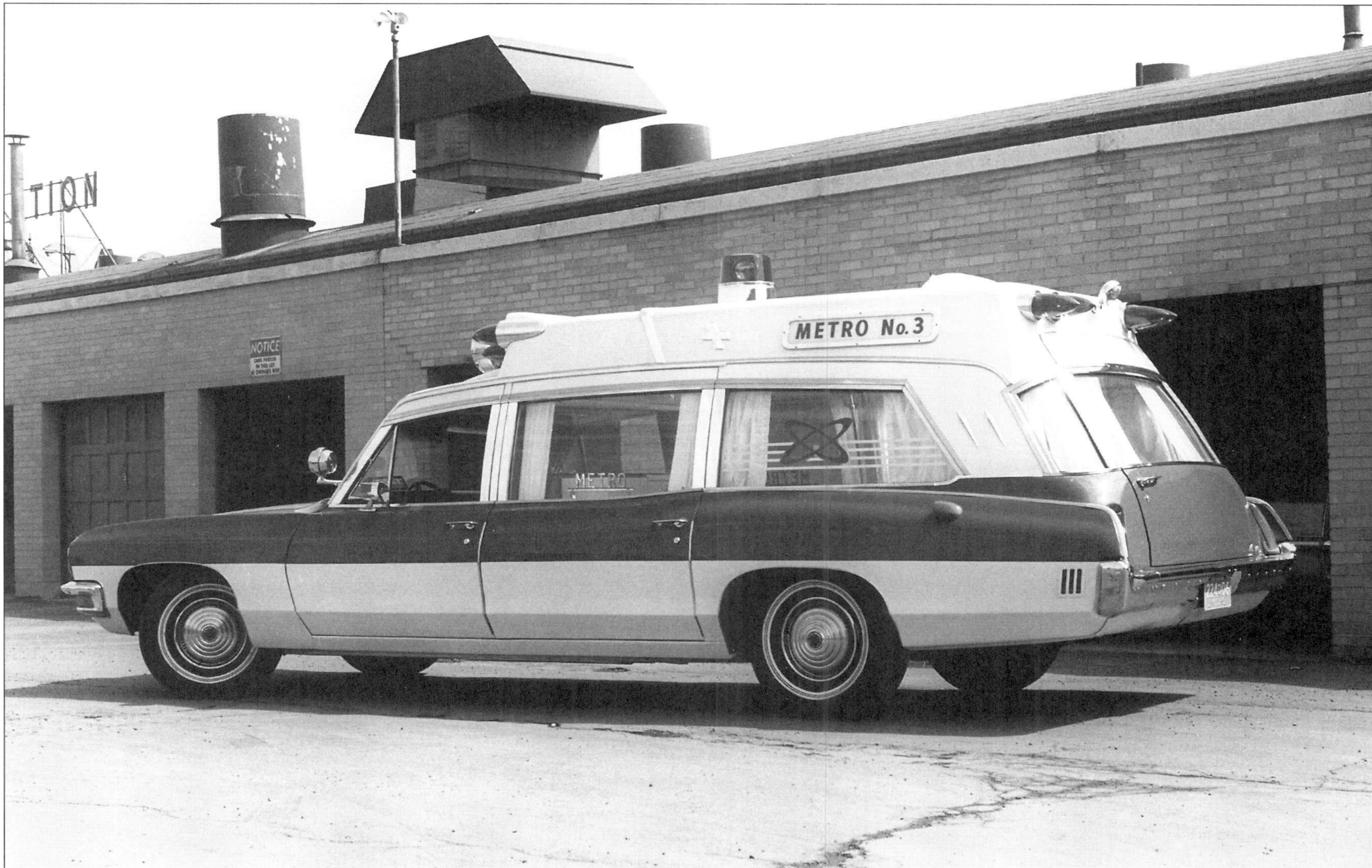

1970 SUPERIOR-PONTIAC MODEL 51-P AMBULANCE - Superior upgraded its long-wheelbase Pontiac ambulance offerings in this year with the addition of the new Model 51-P. The new model designation reflected the car's 51 inches of rear compartment headroom: the "P" indicated a Pontiac. The new Model 51-P used basically the same top structure as Superior's hightop Cadillacs. This 1970 Superior-Pontiac 51-P was photographed in front of the executive garage at the Superior Coach Corp. plant on East Kibby St. in Lima, Ohio.

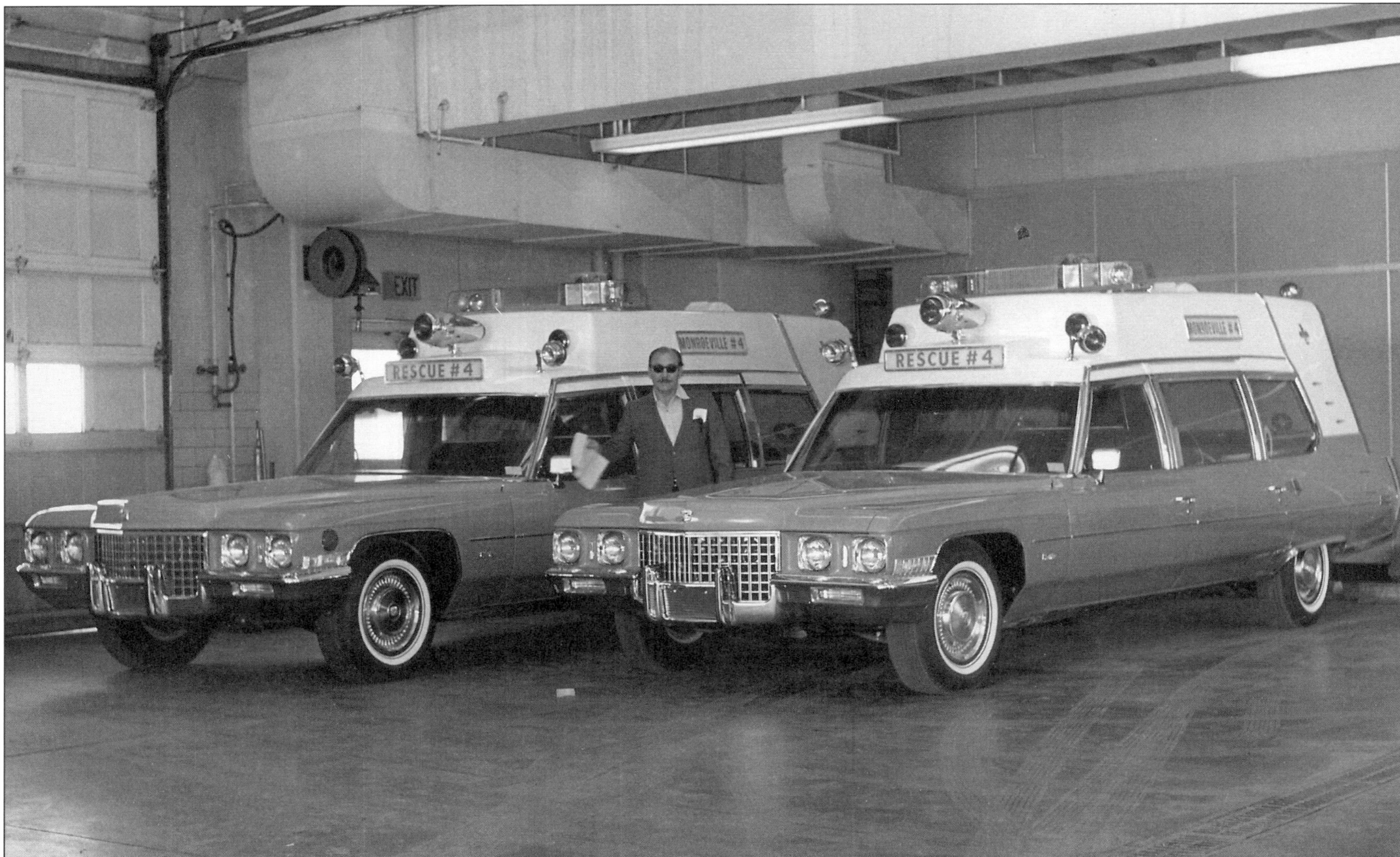

1971 SUPERIOR-CADILLAC MODEL 54 AMBULANCES - Availability of the all-new 1971 Cadillac commercial chassis was seriously delayed by a lengthy strike at General Motors during the last quarter of 1970. Volume production of Superior's extensively redesigned 1971-model professional cars did not begin until early 1971. This photo was taken in the Superior Coach factory driveaway garage in Lima, Ohio. Two brand-new 1971 Superior-Cadillac 54-inch Hightop Ambulances are about to be driven away by members of Rescue Co. No. 4 of Monroeville, Pennsylvania.

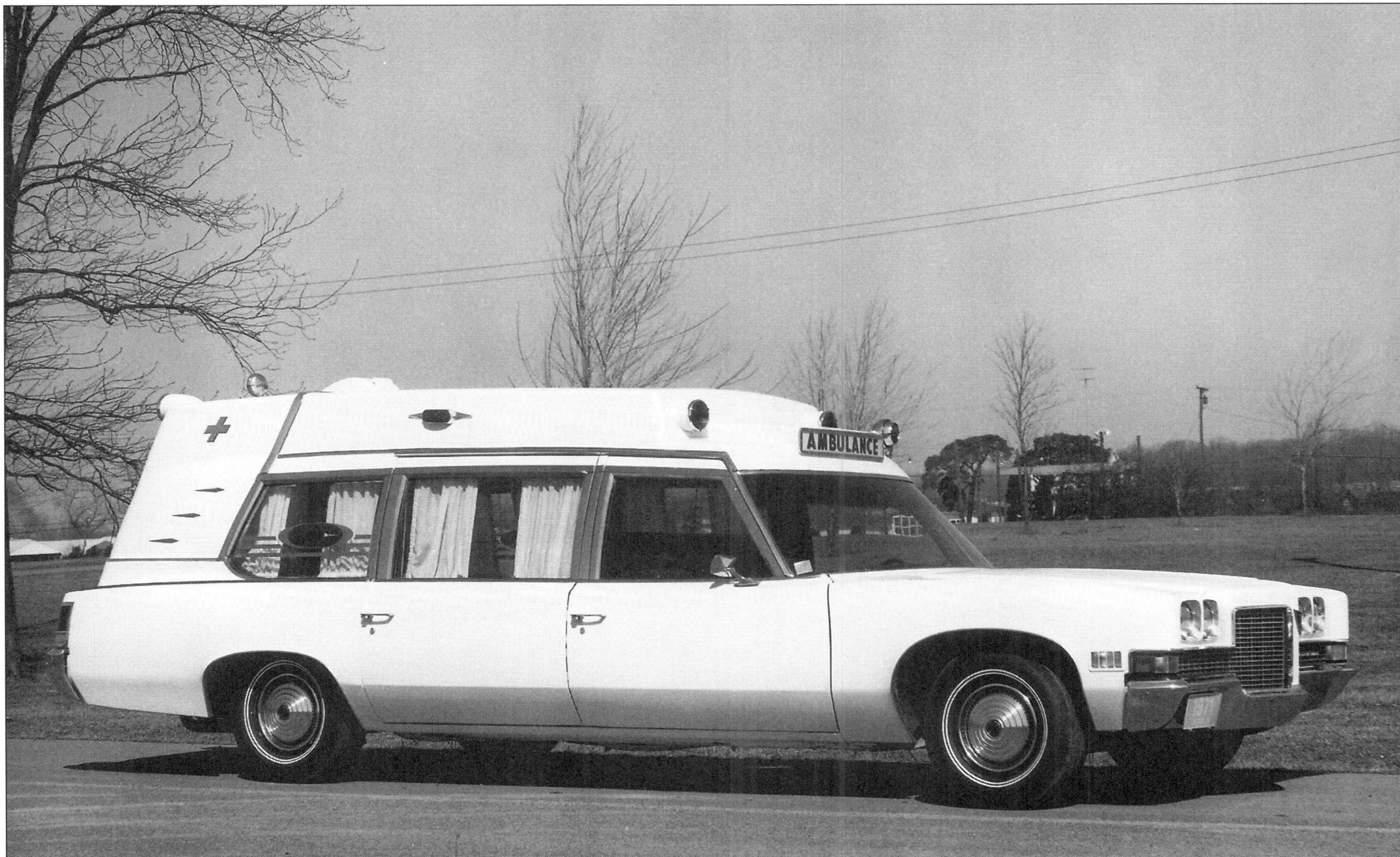

1971 SUPERIOR-PONTIAC 54 AMBULANCE - Superior extensively redesigned both its Cadillac and Pontiac ambulances for 1971. For the first time, Superior's Cadillac and Pontiac ambulances were available with the same high-headroom roof heights. Buyers of Superior-Pontiac ambulances could specify the same 51-inch or 54-inch headroom offered on the company's premium Superior-Cadillac ambulances. This is the 1971 Superior-Pontiac 54. Superior-Pontiacs were also available in standard headroom (41.5-inch) and short-wheelbase Consort versions.

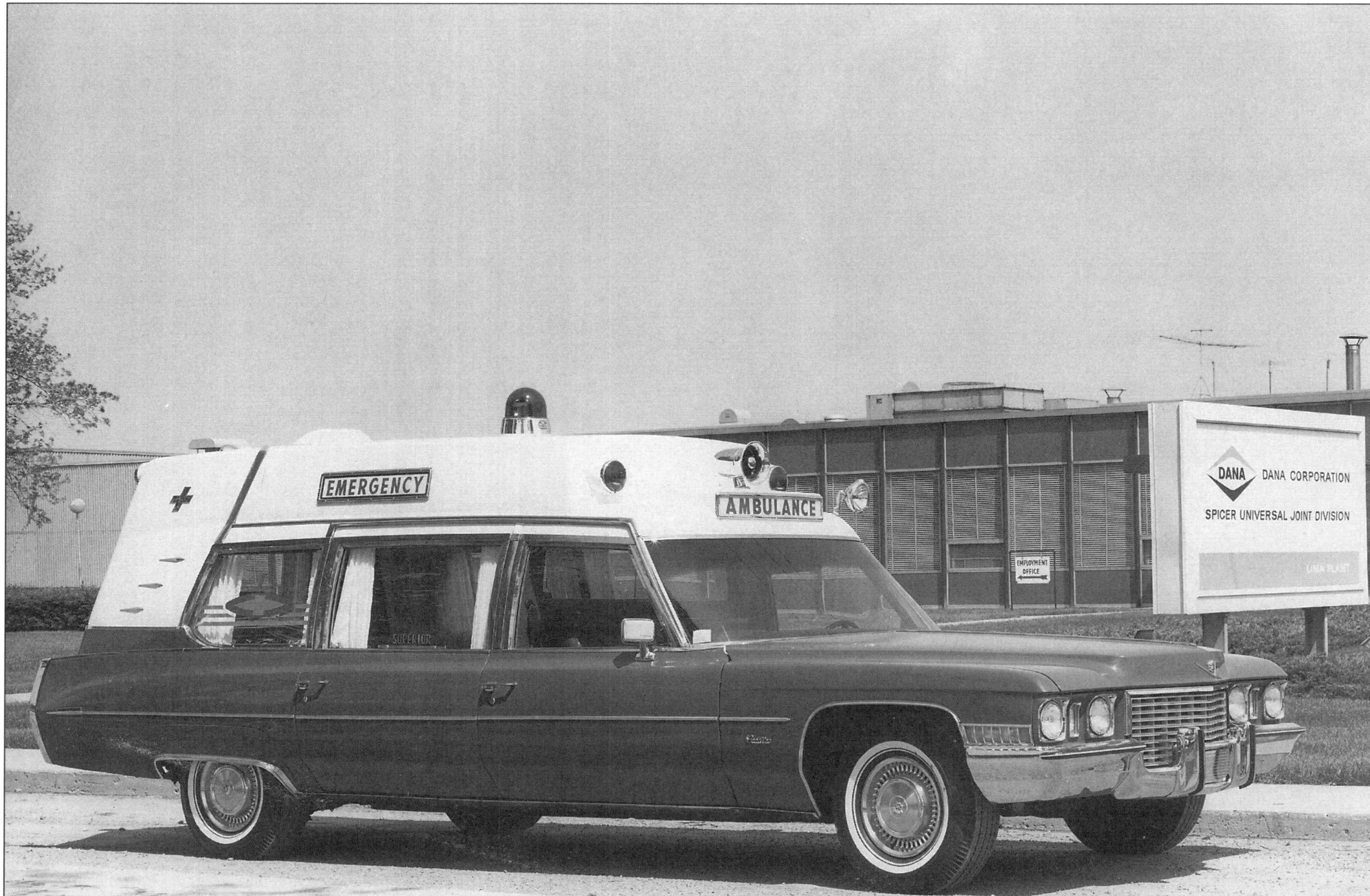

1972 SUPERIOR-CADILLAC 54 HIGHTOP AMBULANCE - Superior Coach celebrated its 50th anniversary in 1972. The most prestigious offering in Superior's Golden Anniversary ambulance lineup was the Superior-Cadillac 54 Hightop. This impressive professional rescue-type ambulance was photographed in front of the Dana Corporation's Spicer Universal Joint Division plant in Lima, Ohio.

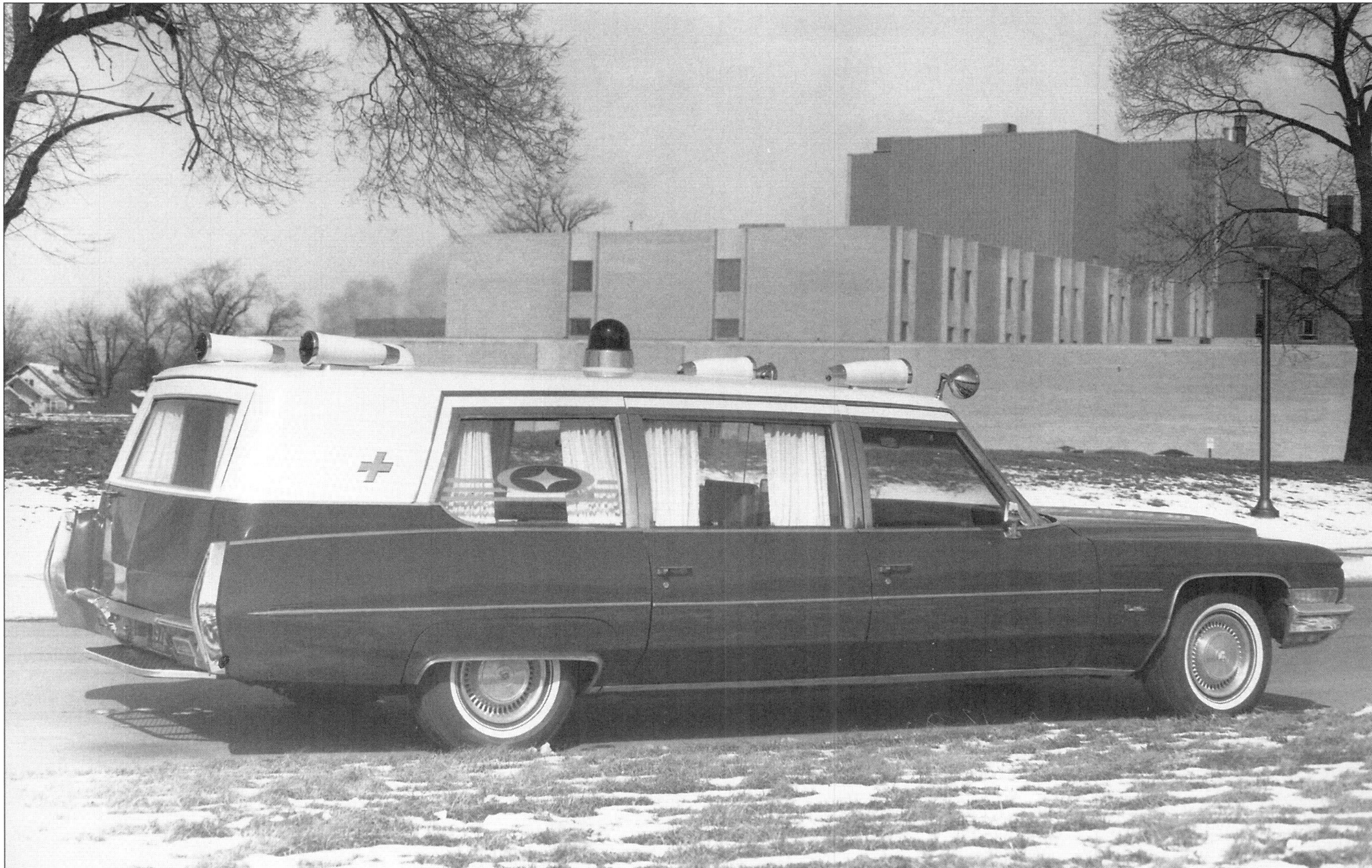

1972 SUPERIOR-CADILLAC SOVEREIGN AMBULANCE - Superior's luxurious Cadillac ambulances were still available with a choice of three roof heights. This is the 41.5-inch standard-headroom model - a 1972 Sovereign in straight ambulance trim. For customers who preferred more rear compartment headroom, Cadillac 51-inch and 54-inch models were available. This Sovereign Ambulance is equipped with four Superior six-inch sealed-beam roof lights and a Federal Beacon Ray.

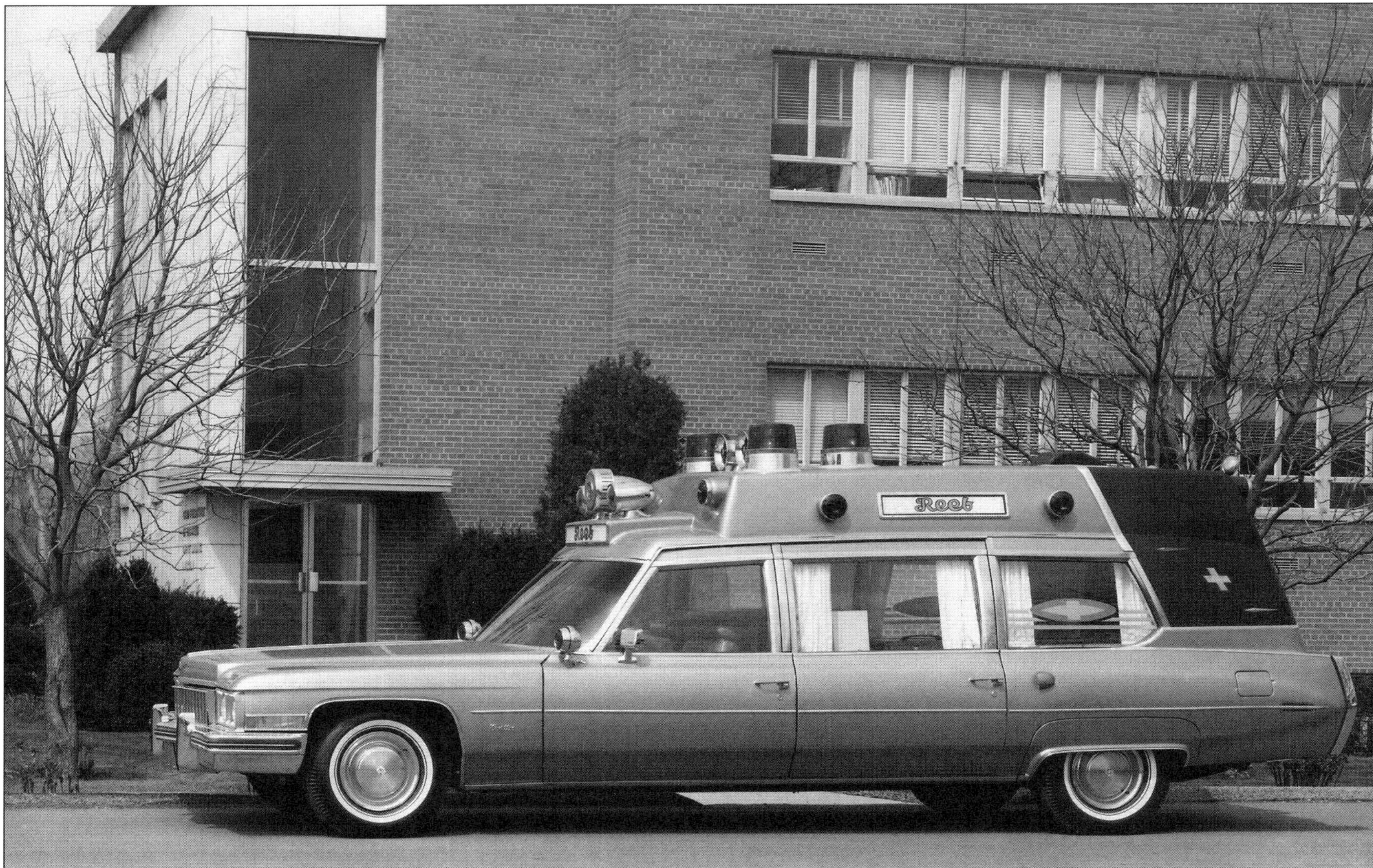

1973 SUPERIOR-CADILLAC 54 AMBULANCE - Some ambulance operators believed strongly in the adage, "see and be seen." The Reeb Funeral Home of Toledo, Ohio, was one such operator. Reeb ran distinctive equipment. Note the black crinkle rear roof area. Reeb's 1973 Superior-Cadillac 54 Ambulance was equipped with *three* flat-top roof beacons, two Solarays, a Federal "Q" siren and a pair of chrome-plated Federal PA electronic siren/speakers.

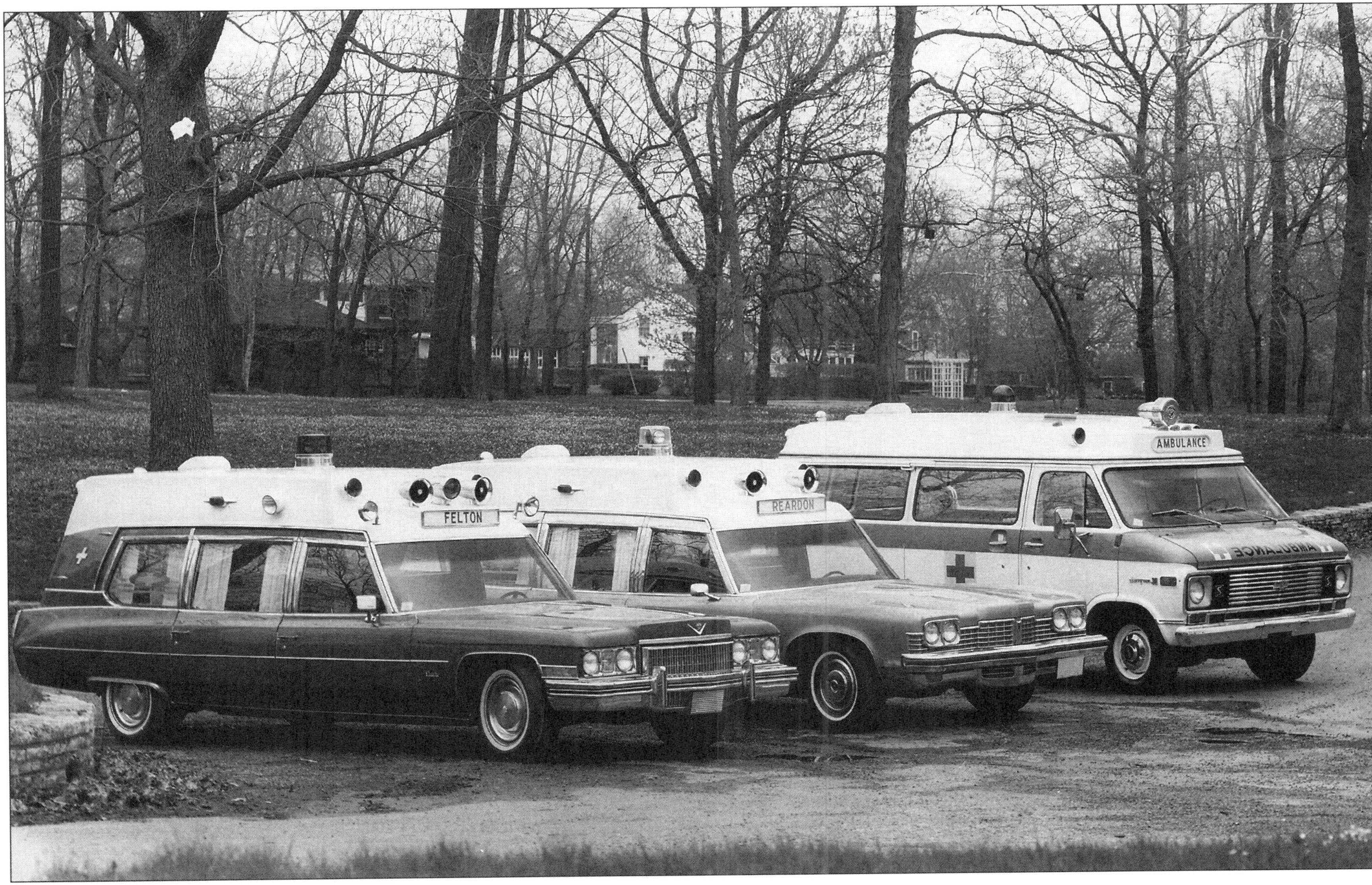

1973 SUPERIOR AMBULANCE FAMILY - To meet the widely varying needs of America's ambulance operators, Superior Coach offered three separate series of ambulances for 1973. From left to right in this family portrait are the flagship 1973 Superior-Cadillac 54 Hightop, Superior-Pontiac 54 Hightop and the new Superior-Chevrolet 61. The Superior 61 was a van conversion with a difference; the Chevy G-30 van was sliced down the middle and widened by 14 inches.

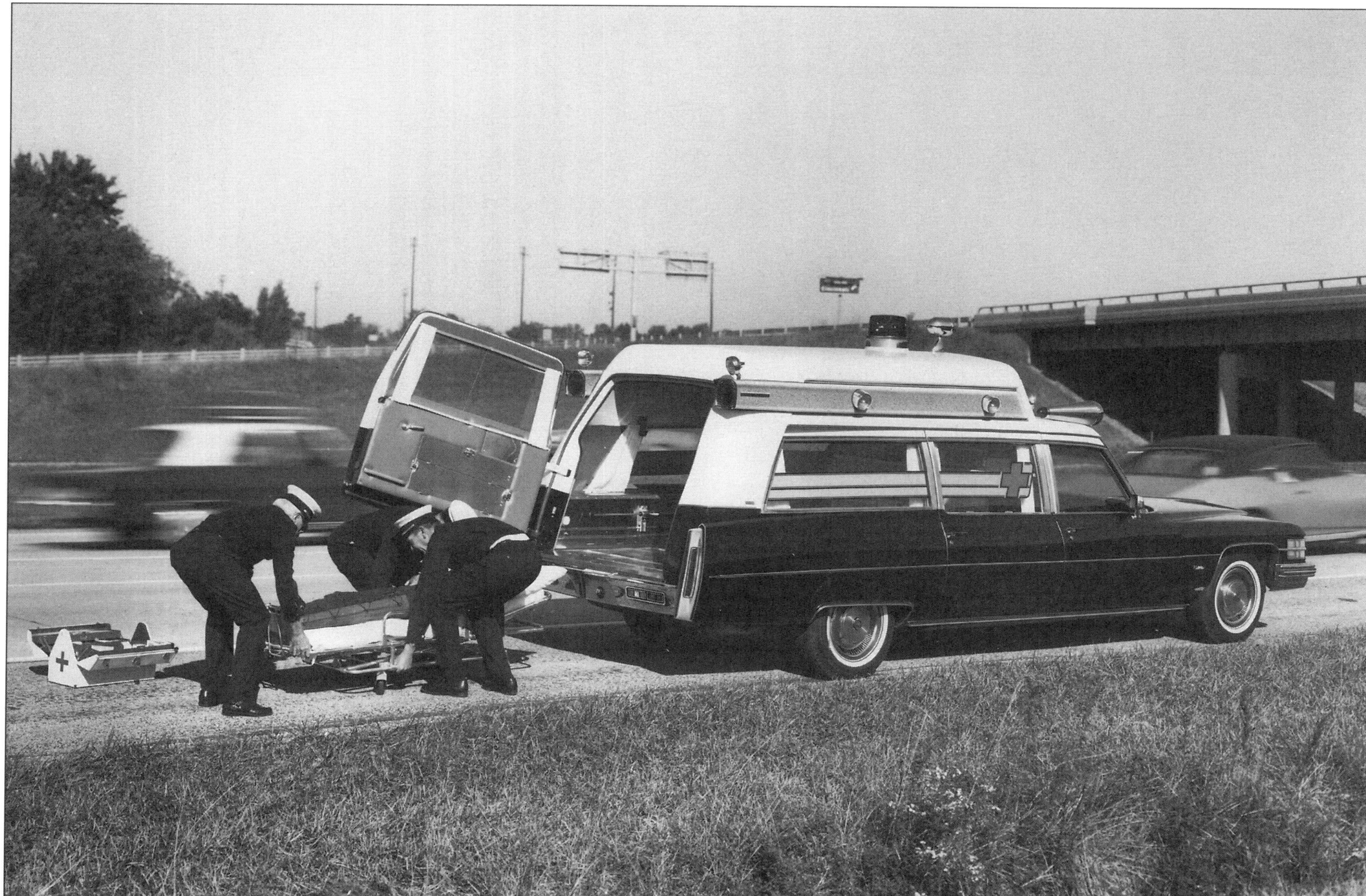

1974 S&S CADILLAC PROFESSIONAL HIGHBODY AMBULANCE - Here's a 1974 S&S Cadillac Professional Ambulance at work. A rescue squad crew prepares to lift a stretcher "patient" into an S&S Cadillac ambulance on a busy freeway near Hess & Eisenhardt's home city of Cincinnati, Ohio. Ambulance manufacturers often posed such scenes for their product catalogs. The highbody Professional was H & E's most prestigious ambulance.

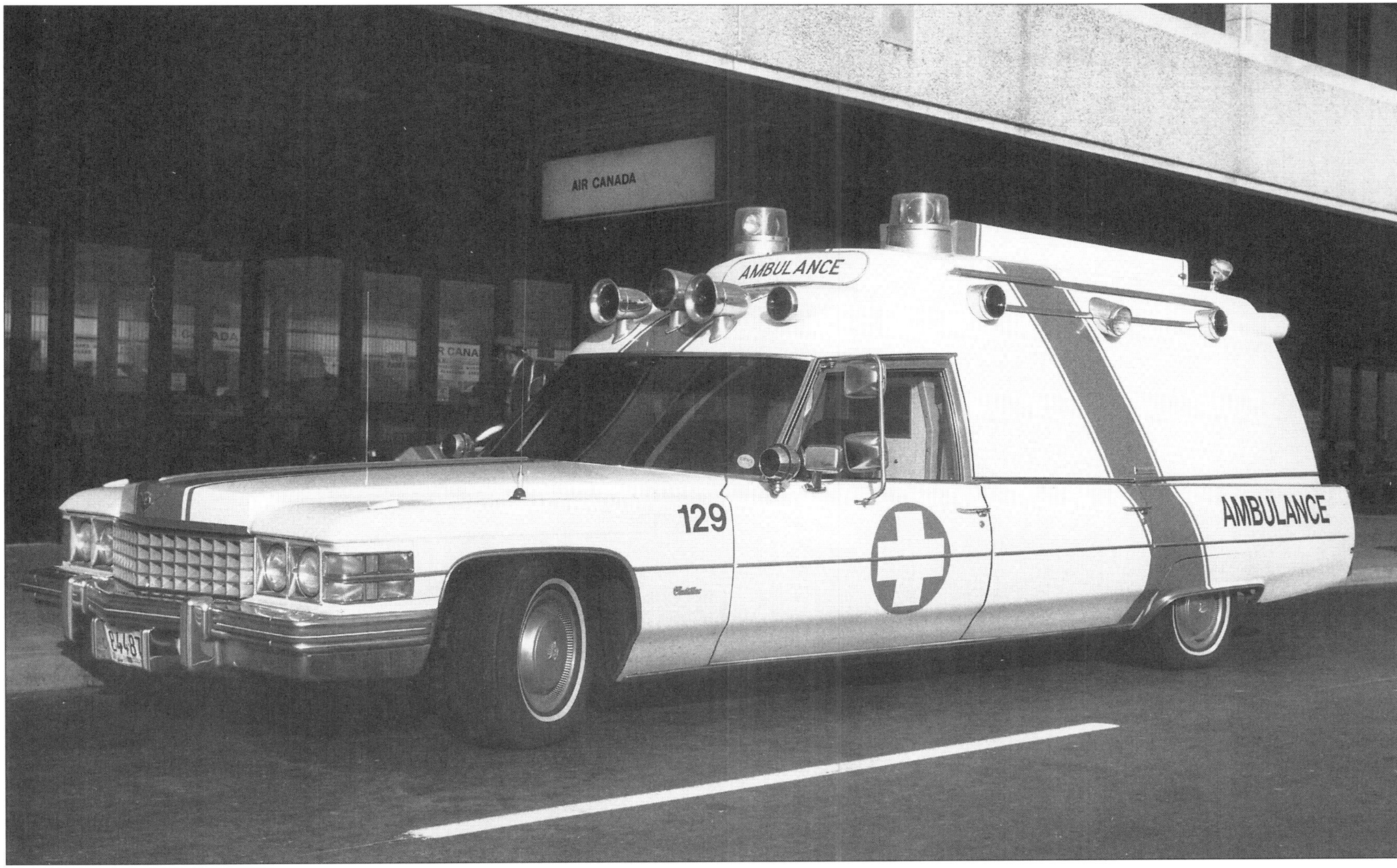

1974 MILLER-METEOR CADILLAC CRITERION RESCUE AMBULANCE - All three of America's major professional car manufacturers — Superior, Miller-Meteor and S&S — had added Cadillac heavy-duty rescue type ambulances to the top of their product lines. Superior offered its hightop 54, S&S its Professional/Medic Mk. 1 and Miller-Meteor its Lifeliner and Criterion. The M/M Criterion had no rear windows on the left side. Author Walt McCall photographed this British Columbia Government unit in front of the Air Canada terminal at Vancouver International Airport.

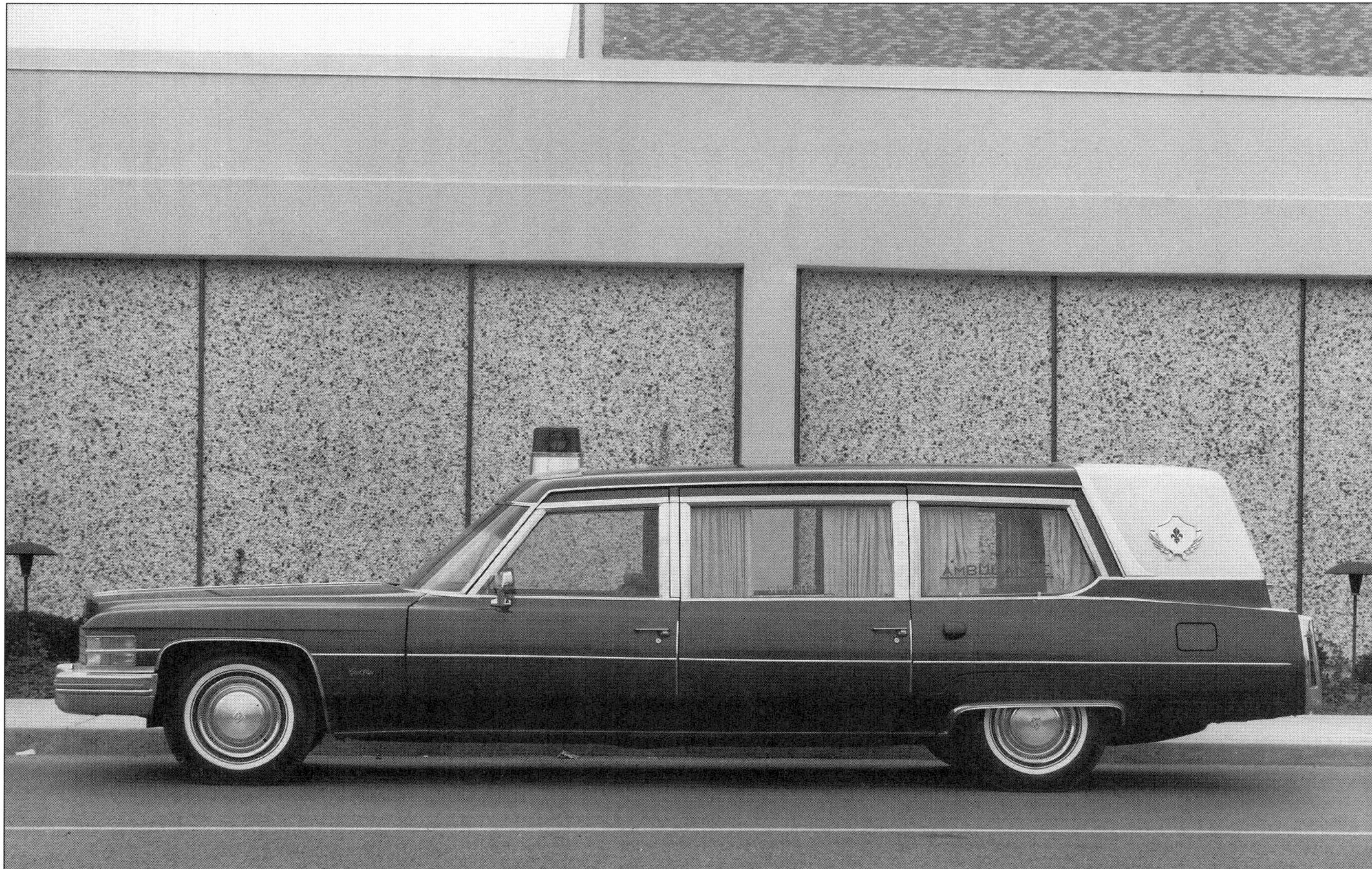

1974 SUPERIOR-CADILLAC CHATEAU BARONET COMBINATION - Superior offered a wide range of Chateau series limousine funeral coaches, combinations and ambulances with some distinctive exterior trim packages. One of these was the "Baronet" package that featured an up-and-over D-pillar roof molding, which gave special definition to the rear roof area. This panel could be ornamented with a large shield emblem. This Chateau Baronet Combination is equipped as an ambulance, with a big flattop roof beacon and "Ambulance" inserts in the rear quarter windows.

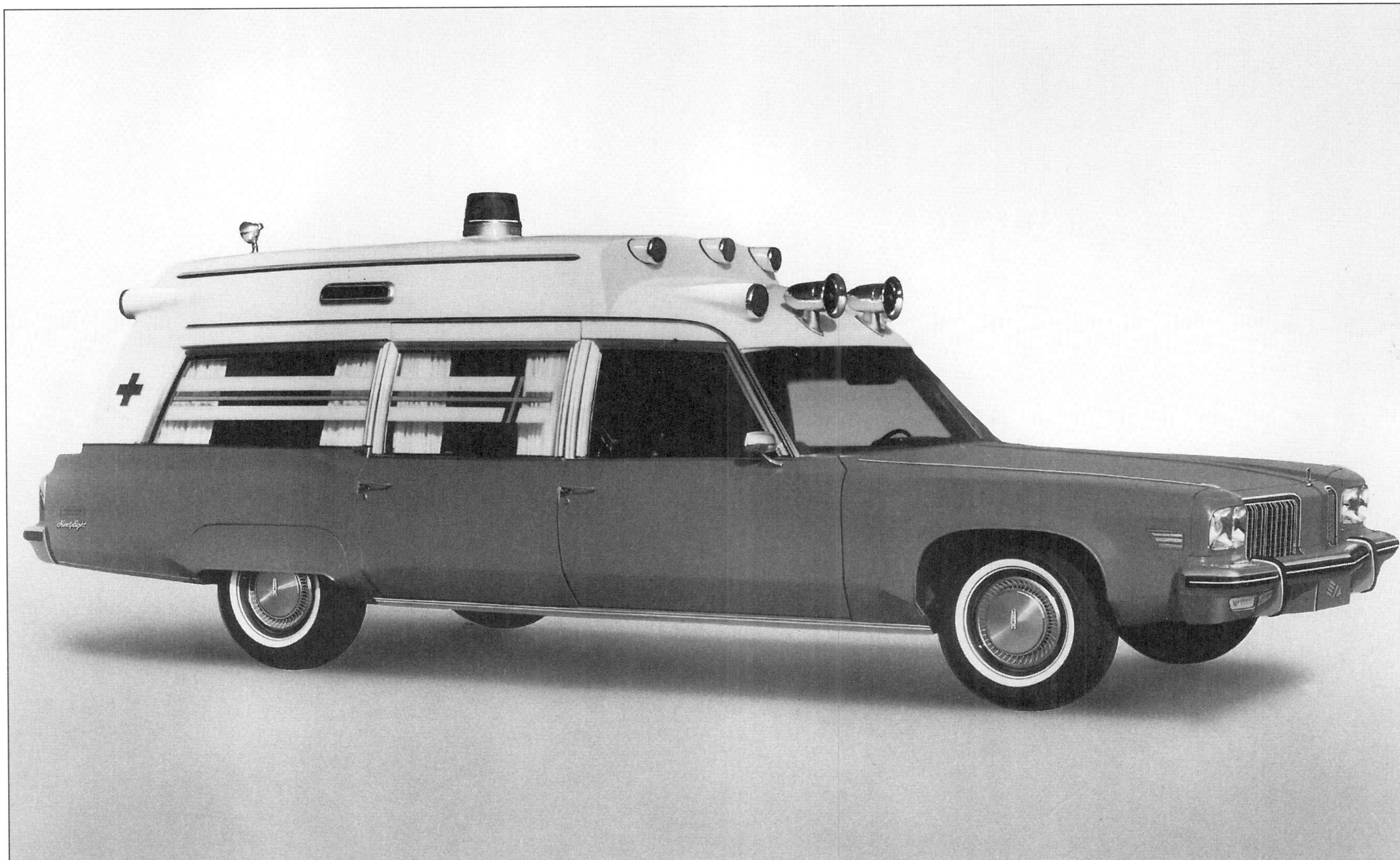

1974 COTNER/BEVINGTON OLDSMOBILE COTINGTON 54 AMBULANCE - Wayne Corporation, which owned Miller-Meteor, had acquired Cotner/Bevington of Blytheville, Arkansas. Wayne's Cotner/Bevington Division continued to build only Oldsmobile-chassis ambulances and funeral coaches, which competed with Superior's Pontiacs. Cotner/Bevington also marketed a compact coach on a standard-wheelbase Oldsmobile chassis called the C/B Seville. Long-wheelbase Cotner/Bevington Oldsmobiles were called Cotingtons. This is a 54-inch hightop ambulance on a 1974 Oldsmobile 98 chassis.

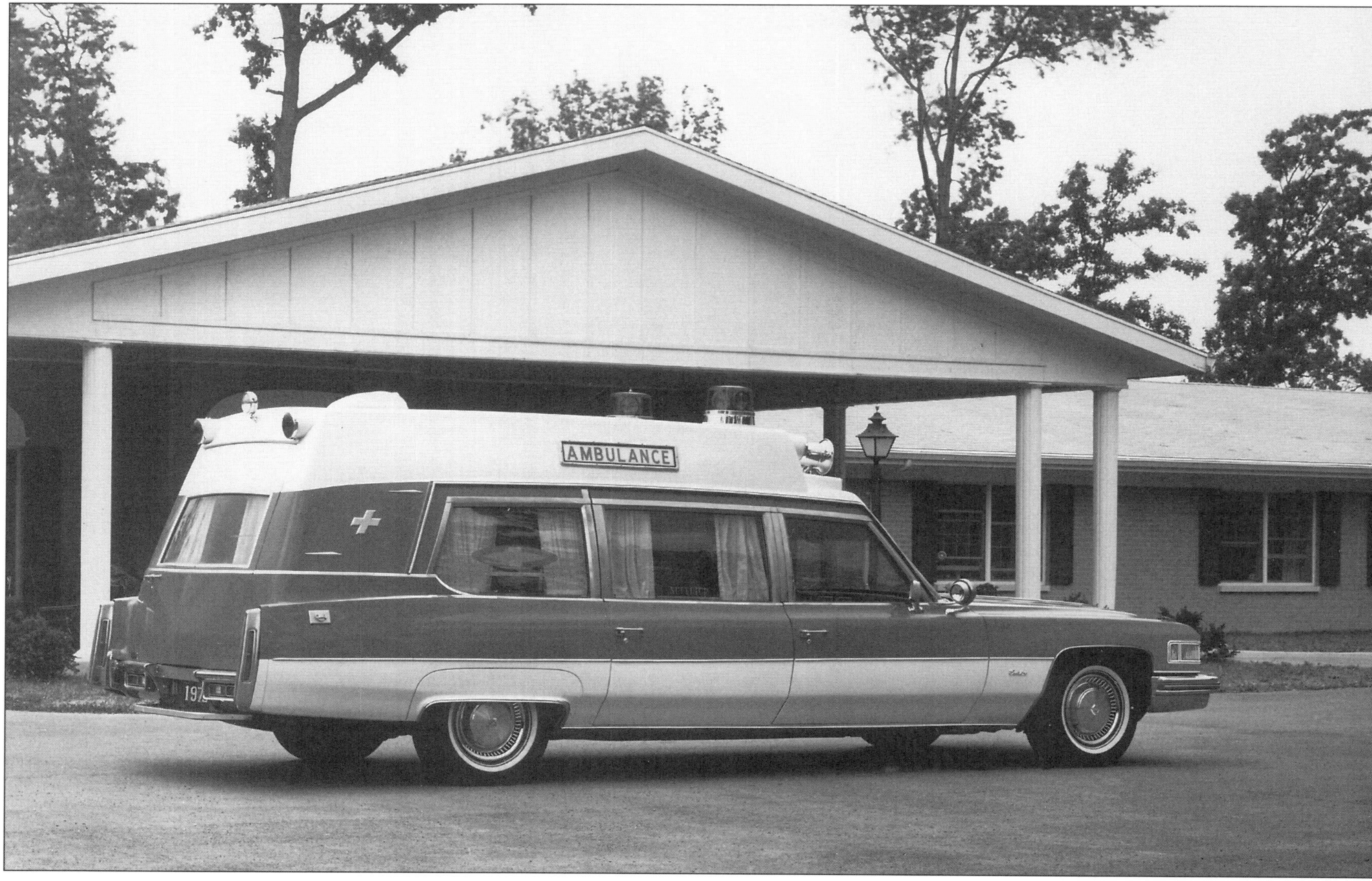

1975 SUPERIOR-CADILLAC 54 AMBULANCE - Superior Coach offered two top-line Cadillac ambulances for 1975: the standard Superior-Cadillac 54 hightop and a new professional rescue model called the 54XL. The XL had blanked-out side windows like Miller-Meteor's Criterion. The Superior-Cadillac 54 offered conventional limousine body styling. These big, expensive Cadillacs complemented the increasingly popular van and modular light truck ambulances now being offered by many manufacturers, including Superior and Wayne Corp.

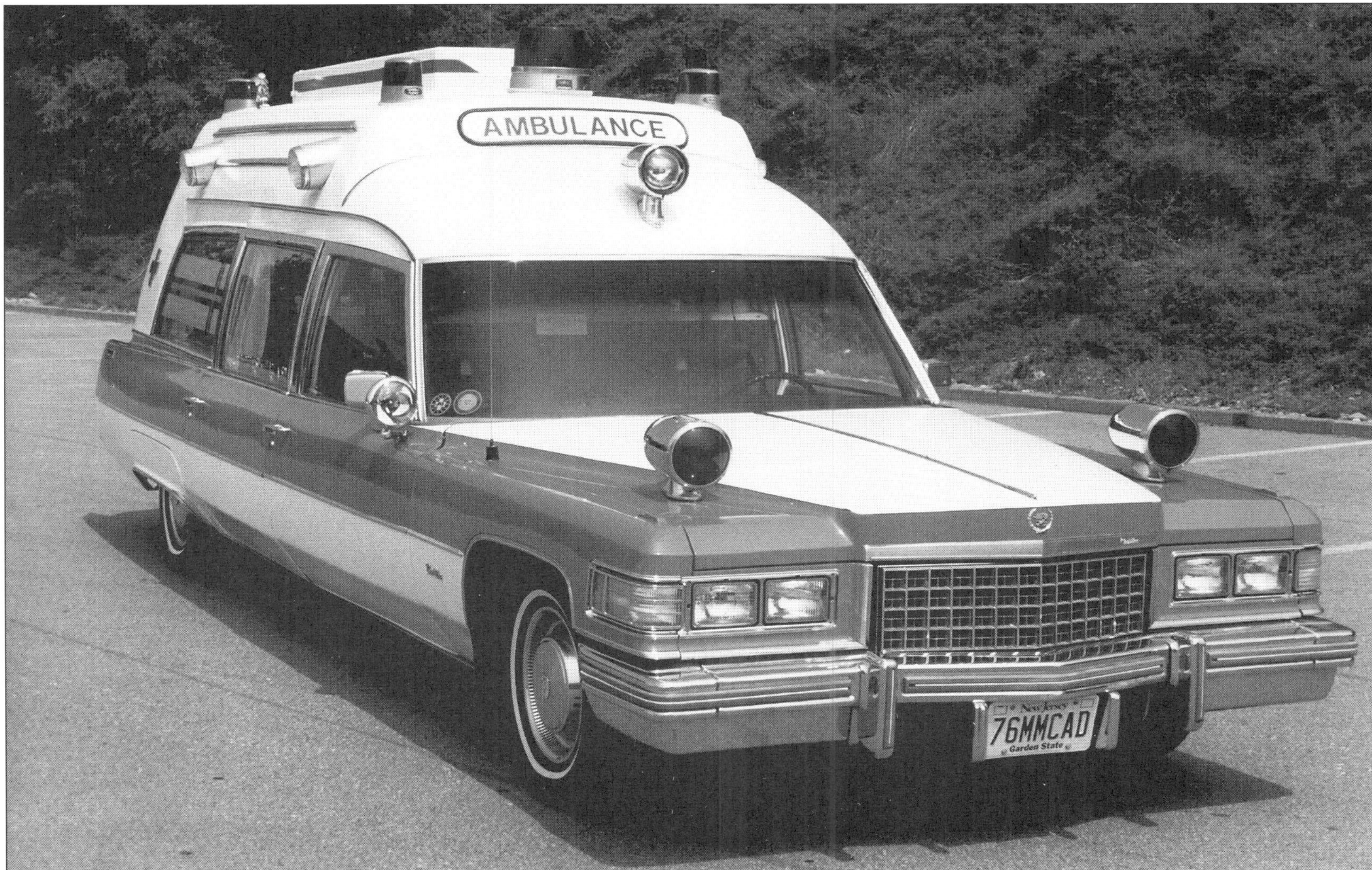

1976 MILLER-METEOR CADILLAC LIFELINER - This would be the last year for the big Cadillac ambulance as we had known it. The writing was already on the wall. Tough new ambulance design regulations were on the way that would all but outlaw passenger car-based ambulances. But the big Cadillac ambulance went out with a bang. Superior, Miller-Meteor and S&S found a large and eager market for the last of the *big* ones. Now owned by Professional Car Society member Craig Stewart of Wood-Ridge, New Jersey, this 1976 Miller-Meteor Cadillac Lifeliner was the last Miller-Meteor ambulance delivered in the state of New Jersey.

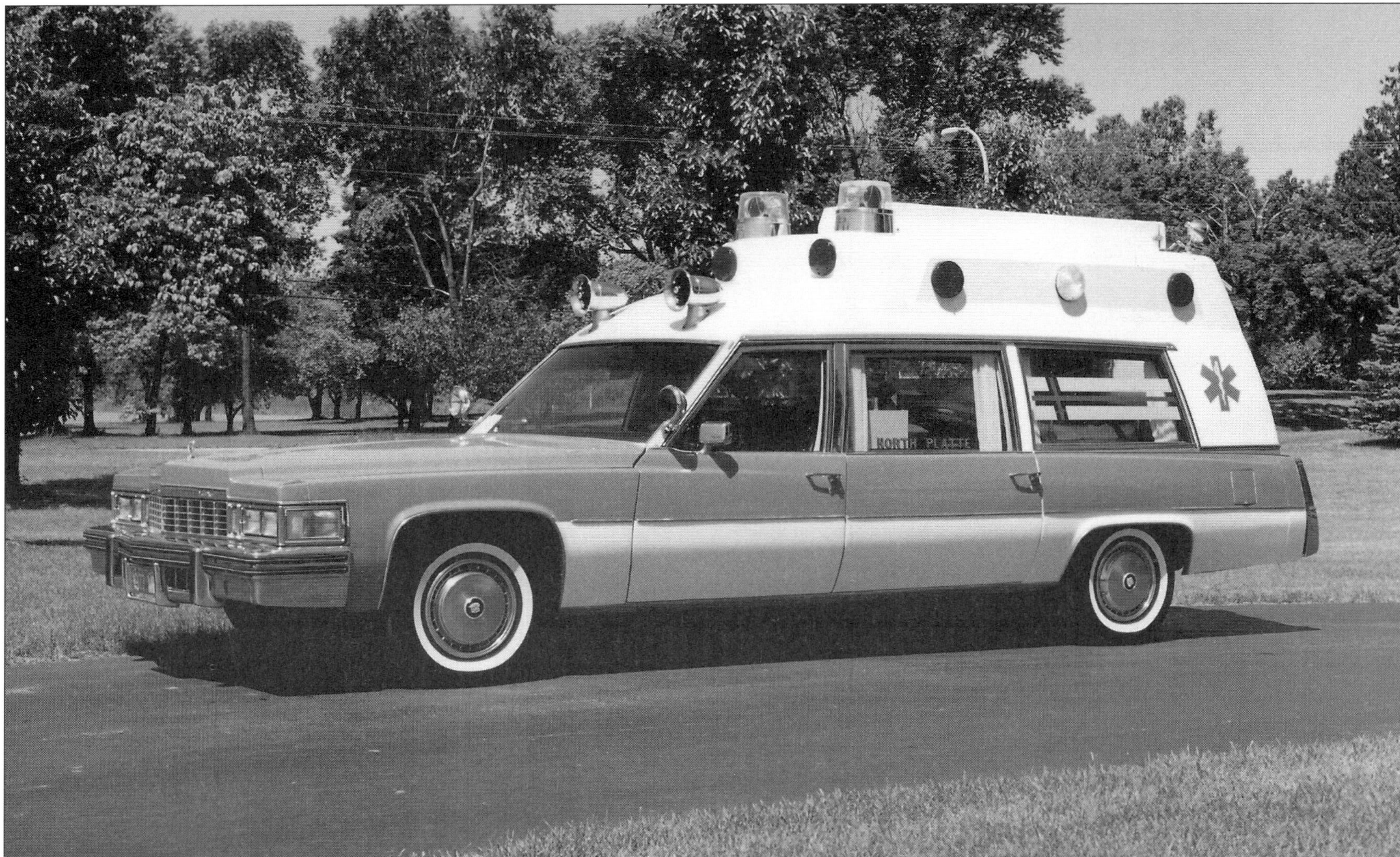

1977 MILLER-METEOR CADILLAC LIFELINER AMBULANCE - The 1977 model year was an epochal one for the American auto industry. To meet stringent new federal fuel economy standards, General Motors "downsized" all of its full-sized 1977 cars, including the Cadillac commercial chassis. The switch to this smaller yet more expensive chassis would have a devastating effect on the U.S. funeral coach and ambulance industry. This 1977 Miller-Meteor Cadillac Lifeliner, which saw service in North Platte, North Dakota is now owned by Warren Waterman of Taylor, Michigan.

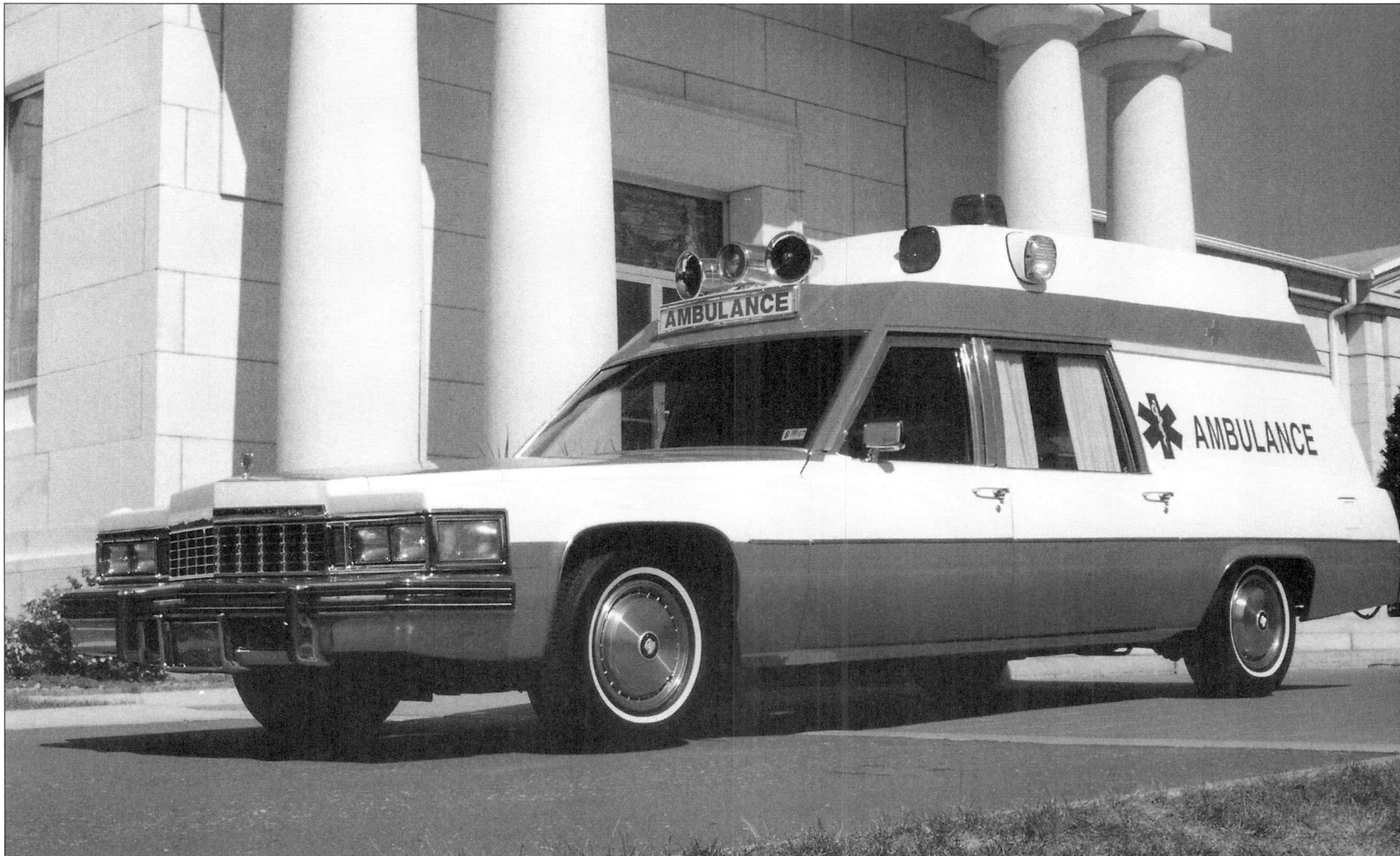

1977 SUPERIOR-CADILLAC TRANSPORT AMBULANCE - Superior built only ten Cadillac ambulances in each of the 1977, 1978 and 1979 model years. Introducing them much later than the company's downsized funeral cars, Superior called its all-new smaller hightop the Superior Transport Ambulance — a name which implied patient *transfer* rather than emergency response service, just like the single-purpose "Invalid" ambulances built much earlier in the century. This 1977 Superior-Cadillac is owned by Professional Car Society member Mike Barruzza of Bristol, Pennsylvania.

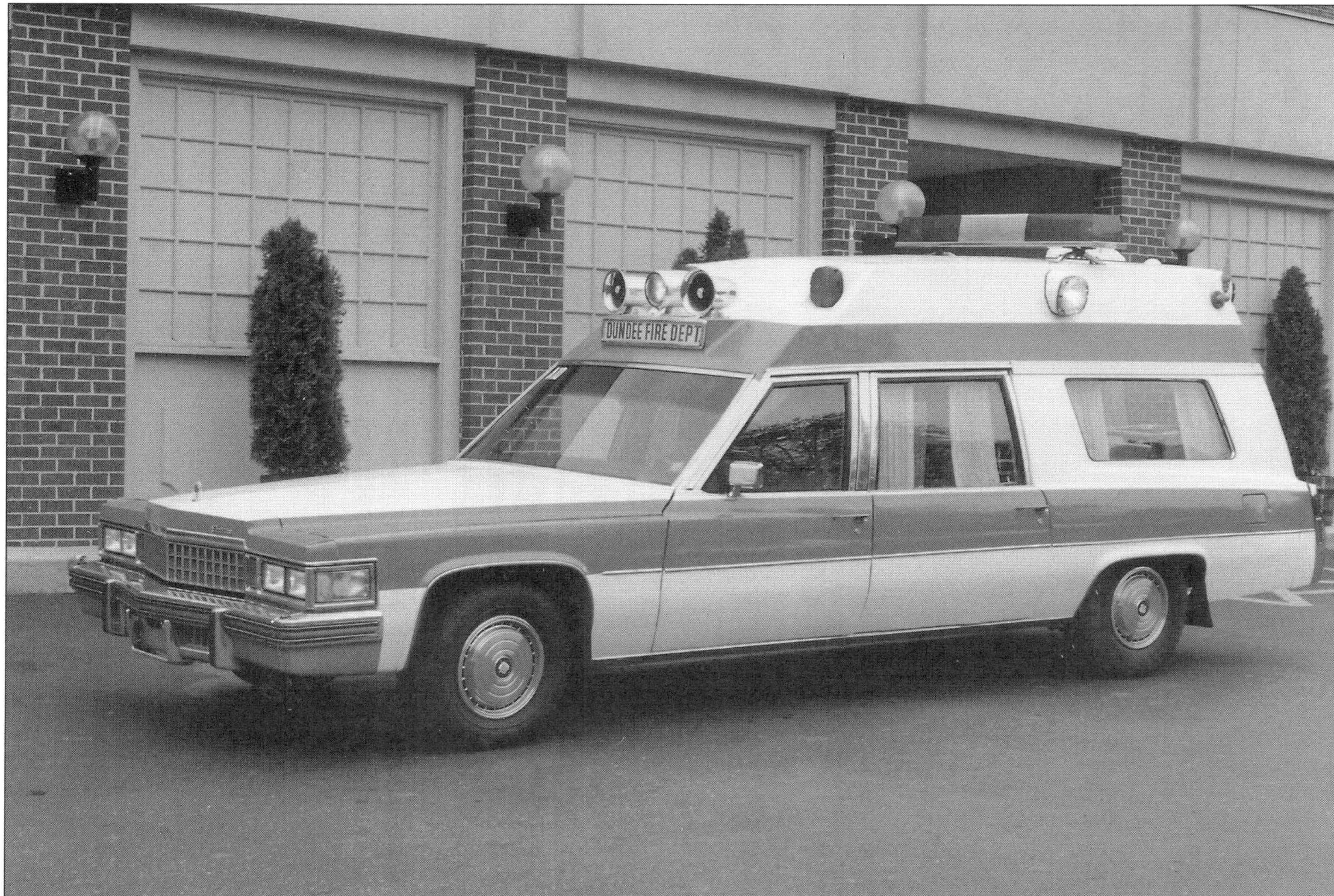

1978 SUPERIOR-CADILLAC TRANSPORT AMBULANCE - The curtain was coming down on the passenger car-type ambulance. Cadillac ambulance production had dwindled to a trickle at Superior and Miller-Meteor. Hess & Eisenhardt had ceased production of S&S ambulances at the end of the 1976 model year. Miller-Meteor built only four 1978 Cadillac ambulances, its last year of ambulance production. The Village of Dundee, New York, purchased this 1978 Superior-Cadillac Transport Ambulance. Note the rear-mounted roof light bar.

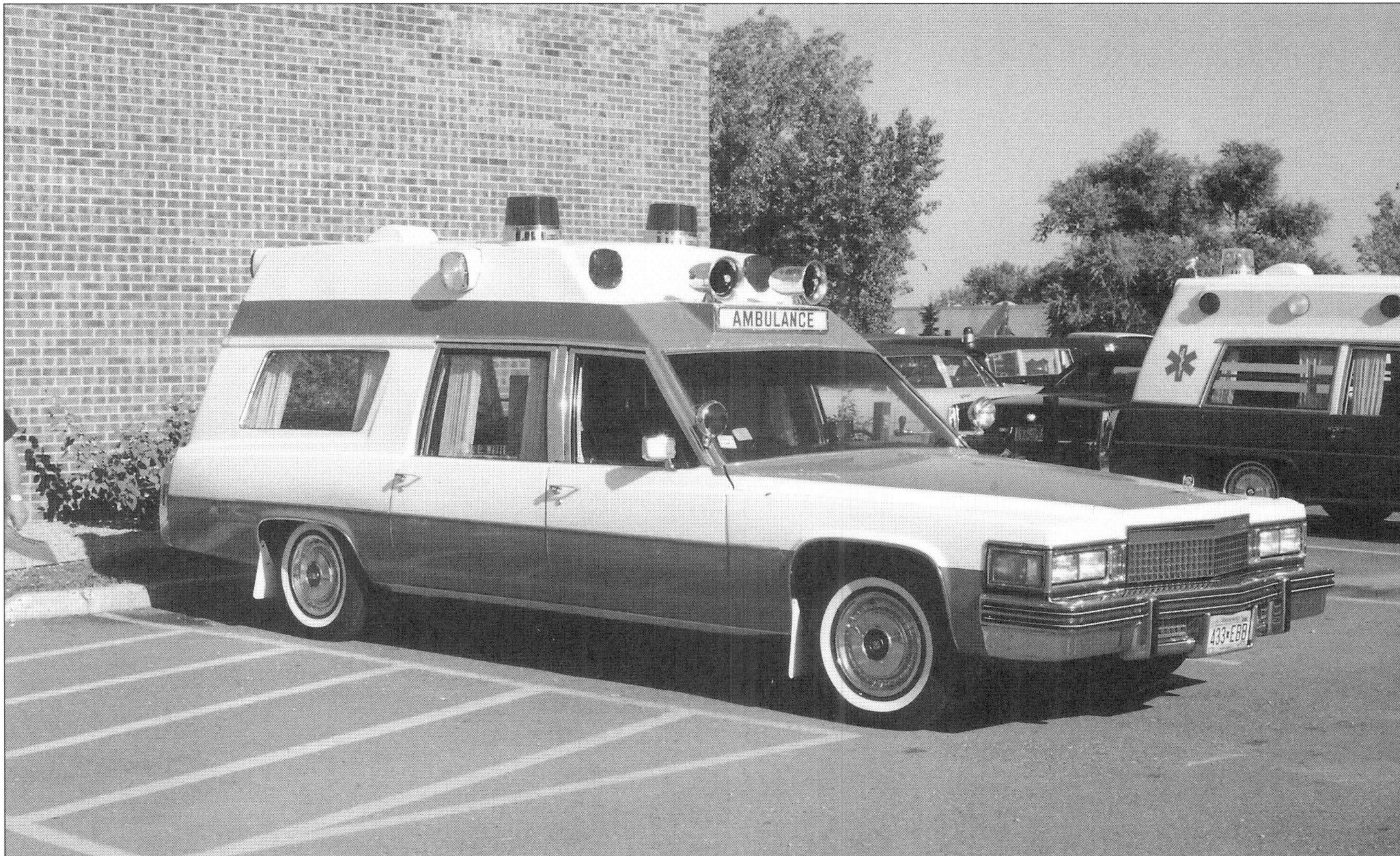

1979 SUPERIOR-CADILLAC TRANSPORT AMBULANCE - A long and distinguished chapter in American ambulance history ended when Superior built the last Cadillac ambulance in America at the end of the 1979 model year. The last Cadillac ambulance was purchased by Dr. Roger D. White of the Mayo Clinic who had headed a spirited, if unsuccessful, campaign to save the passenger car-based ambulance from extinction. Dr. White lovingly maintains his 1979 Superior, which is a regular participant at Professional Car Society meets in the Midwest. This photo was taken at the 1996 PCS International Meet in St. Paul, Minnesota.

Bibliography

McPherson, Thomas A., FLXIBLE PROFESSIONAL VEHICLES: THE COMPLETE HISTORY, Specialty Vehicle Press, Don Mills, Ontario, Canada 1993.

McPherson, Thomas A., THE EUREKA COMPANY; A COMPLETTE HISTORY, Specialty Vehicle Press, Don Mills, Ontario, Canada 1994.

McPherson, Thomas A., SUPERIOR; THE COMPLETE HISTORY, Specialty Vehicle Press, Don Mills, Ontario, Canada 1995.

McPherson, Thomas A., AMERICAN FUNERAL CARS & AMBULANCES, Crestline Publishing, Glen Ellyn, Illinois 1973.

McCall, Walter M. P., McCall, Editor - THE PROFESSIONAL CAR, quarterly magazine of the Professional Car Society, Columbus Ohio.